Fundamentals of Eye Training

1. Vision can be improved by natural methods.

2. Tension causes eye strain and impairs vision. Relaxation relieves tension.

3. Relaxed eyes are normal eyes. When eyes lose their relaxation and become tense, they strain and stare and the vision becomes poor.

4. Vision can be improved only by education in proper seeing. Proper seeing is relaxed seeing. Normal eyes shift rapidly and continuously. Eyes with defective vision are fixed and staring. When staring eyes learn to shift, vision is improved.

5. The eyeball is like the camera, and changes in focal length. To focus the camera, you must adjust the distance from the negative to the front of the camera.

PAPERBACK
EXCHANGE
131 Vesta
Reno, Nevada 89502
WE SELL - WE TRADE

Reading Page

c a i g

m e f t s

t p j x n q

l w r y s u a

e v g p c f d t

k a b e n e m y

b g p l a i q d o

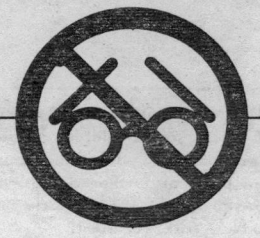

A REMARKABLE TECHNIQUE TO RESTORE YOUR EYESIGHT!

12 WEEKS TO BETTER VISION

by Barbara Hughes

PINNACLE BOOKS   NEW YORK

ATTENTION: SCHOOLS AND CORPORATIONS

PINNACLE Books are available at quantity discounts with bulk purchases for educational, business or special promotional use. For further details, please write to: SPECIAL SALES MANAGER, Pinnacle Books, Inc., 1430 Broadway, New York, NY 10018.

WRITE FOR OUR FREE CATALOG

If there is a Pinnacle Book you want—and you cannot find it locally—it is available from us simply by sending the title and price plus 75¢ to cover mailing and handling costs to:

>Pinnacle Books, Inc.
>Reader Service Department
>1430 Broadway
>New York, NY 10018

Please allow 6 weeks for delivery.

_____Check here if you want to receive our catalog regularly.

---

12 WEEKS TO BETTER VISION

Copyright © 1981 by Barbara Hughes

All rights reserved, including the right to reproduce this book or portions thereof in any form.

An original Pinnacle Books edition, published for the first time anywhere.

First printing, August 1981
Second printing, December 1981

ISBN: 0-523-41032-8

Printed in the United States of America

PINNACLE BOOKS, INC.
1430 Broadway
New York, New York 10018

For my teacher,
Janet Goodrich

CONTENTS

Introduction
1. A Way of Looking at Seeing
2. William H. Bates, Vision-ary
3. Seeing and Vision
4. In-sight: Mind and Vision
5. Seeing Is Believing
6. Let's See . . .
7. The Common Disorders: Nearsighted, Farsighted, Astigmatic, Middle-aged Sight
8. For More Serious Disorders: Ambliopia, Squint, Cataracts, Detached Retina, Glaucoma, Night Blindness
9. Working with Children
10. The Bates Laws of Vision

INTRODUCTION

Can you imagine breaking your leg and having your doctor give you crutches to use for the rest of your life? Imagine being told by this same doctor that your leg would get worse and worse in spite of these crutches? You think that is crazy? No, you don't. For in fact, every *minute* many Americans visit such doctors, who not only tell us that but prescribe the crutches as well! And we pay for the service. Even thank them. Except instead of broken legs, it is for eyes. And the crutches are glasses. You don't think so? Read on. See for yourself.

Thirty years ago, in the fifth grade, I began having trouble seeing the blackboard. I had always sat in the back of the classroom, where I could get away with talking or passing notes once in a while, but now I had to move up to the second row, where such maneuvers were no longer possible. My compensation, I thought at the time, was that I would get to wear glasses like my older sister. But, oddly, my parents did not believe I needed glasses, and no one at school bothered to test me. (I report all this not out of nostalgia but because I shall refer back to it later on in the book.) By seventh grade, however, my defect had become obvious, so I now got to fulfill my wish to be like my sister. Unfortunately, the reality was not what I had expected. I now had the proverbial "four eyes" to add to my prepubescent charm, a pair of pinkish plastic-framed glasses that permitted me to see everyone's skin problems with crisp accuracy. But what did I know? I was a kid. Half the world wore glasses. Besides, the doctor was right: my eyes got progressively worse.

Twenty-five years later, on a warm summer day in Los Angeles, I had an experience that would turn my whole way of thinking completely around. It was a tiny enough event, seemingly random, but its smallness proved to be the smallness of a seed. I sat reading in our living room, facing a large picture window that overlooked our garden. For some reason, I looked up from my book, then slipped off my glasses. This was something I never did because my visual acuity then measured 10/400, which means that what a person with normal vision could see from 400 feet away, I could see only from 10 feet or closer. So what I saw out in front of me that day was a bright blur in which objects lost their edges and melted into one another. But as I gazed into the haze, I had this thought: *I don't want to see like this anymore. I'm going to do something about it.* I put on my glasses, and the next thought seemed to erase the first: *So what can you do about it?* I went back to my book and had no further thoughts about the matter until two days later, when I picked up my daughter from school. She needed a book; we would pass a bookstore on the way home. Books are a weakness of mine, but with a library filled with many unread volumes, I needed another book the way my daughter needed another hot dog. So to forestall my own addiction, I asked the clerk to find the one my daughter needed. I merely gazed at the spines of the other books that stood on the shelf where he was looking. I was determined: I would not buy another book. But a title jumped out at me—*Do You Really Need Eyeglasses?* I suddenly recalled my forlorn little self-assertion of two days previous: *I don't want to see like this anymore. I'm going to do something about it.* My resolve broke and I bought the book. I've never been sorry.

The book quickly led to frustration. First, because I wanted a miracle; second, because the instructions were not that clearly written. But, once aroused, I'm hard to stop. I checked the Yellow Pages, found a special listing—"Vision Training"—and called the one person who called herself the Bates-Corbett Training Center. When she did not want to see me because of her schedule, I simply refused to take no for an answer. She gave in, and with great excitement, I went to my first lesson.

Janet Goodrich, my teacher, advised me to get a 20/40 glasses correction. Normally, when you get glasses, you get a 20/20 correction so that you can see at 20 feet what the supposedly normal person also sees at 20 feet but without the glasses. A 20/40 prescription would mean that there would be some blur, though not very much. Janet explained that such lenses would give me some flexibility as my vision improved with the exercises. If I wore a 20/20 correction, she explained, my eyes would have to *adjust* to that correction; with 20/40 lenses, I would have some room to maintain any minor improvement I made. She also advised me that the Bates techniques were not eye exercises, as I called them, but relaxation exercises that result in visual improvement.

My doctor looked just a little skeptical when I explained all this to him—in other words, he masked his amusement at this screwy lady—and guessed that my eyes might make a tiny improvement as a result of relaxation techniques. But "tiny" was all he'd allow.

"Why, if you can improve your eyes even halfway," he said magnanimously, "I'll write it up in one of the major ophthalmological journals."

He was a man I respected—a doctor, a man of scientific background and philosophy, an eye surgeon known and respected in his field. If my respect and blind faith in doctors in general had not been seriously undermined over the years, I probably would have stopped right there. But I had had sufficient experience with too many of these men of so-called scientific method, who practiced medicine like priests instead of scientists, as petty demagogues instead of thinkers, who represented the backwaters of traditional knowledge rather than the lifestream of investigation and development. And I had had enough. Doctors had lost their power and mystique. I had known for some time that I was on my own, so I took the good doctor's irony as a challenge.

A year later, I returned to him. From my previous visit's measurement of 10/400, I now measured 20/100. Amazingly enough, the doctor seemed to have forgotten his proposal. He didn't breathe a word about a major ophthalmological journal. Because he was an acquaintance of my husband, I politely refrained from reminding him of his offer, which I had innocently believed he would be delighted to fulfill. When the appointment was over, I left his office thrilled to know I had improved my vision more than halfway, but also cynical, realizing what a man had to do to protect his career.

He was not even curious. Or surprised. He did not ask a single question! For the rest of the day, he fitted people with glasses. They thanked him. They paid him. And all those people are out there somewhere, wearing those crutches that offer them the sole benefit of seeing other people's skin problems clearly. Sure, they will see more than that. But their vision will deteriorate. The doctor will give them new glasses. And for what? Is it really necessary?

See for yourself that vision is not what you were

taught, that it *can* be improved, even completely corrected, given no serious abnormality of the eye, optic nerve, or brain; but you will also see for yourself with your own eyes, without glasses. Because we are so well trained to accept books as authoritative, I have deliberately included views from a variety of sources. The journal entries are taken from my own journal over the period of time I was working on regaining my vision. I have included these to show the many stages I went through on my own path toward clearer vision: sometimes I made absurd mistakes; sometimes I had wonderful flashes of insight. The sources of the other entries are clearly identified. Some are Bates sources—Aldous Huxley, Bates himself, Margaret Corbett; others are non-Bates. Don't simply accept the Bates point of view. Read the varying opinions. Truly see for yourself.

CHAPTER 1
A way of looking at seeing

What is vision? This question is central to the whole issue we are examining because a major portion of our knowledge and information in life comes to us through the visual sense. But perhaps more significant is the fact that your definition of vision will reveal how you think about your body and the power you do or do not have over it. Your definition will also reflect your beliefs about vision, which, in turn, will affect your vision itself. So look at it. What is vision?

The traditional view offered to us by the science of ophthalmology is that vision is the act of perceiving the world through the eyes. The interesting point here is that the emphasis is on *eyes*. When our vision blurs, we go to a doctor to have our eyes examined. We are told after the exam that we are nearsighted or farsighted, getting old, or have astigmatism—these being the most common vision "disorders." If we ask what nearsighted or farsighted means, we are told that the eyeball is too long, or too short, so that the image of what we are looking at does not fall on the part of the retina that "sees" best (see Diagrams 1 and 2). So what is wrong with our vision is to be found in the *eyes*. "Getting old" means we are in our forties or fifties, and the lens just inside the eyeball is getting hard as a result of the aging process. Astgmatism is described as a condition in

Diagram #1

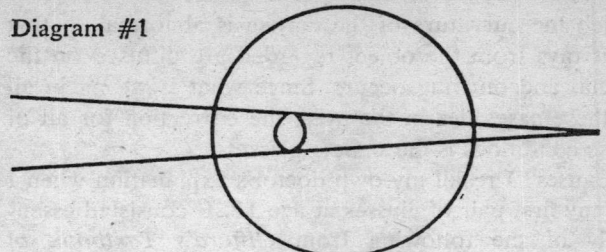

The hyperopic eye (farsighted eye)
The light rays fall behind the retina.

Diagram #2

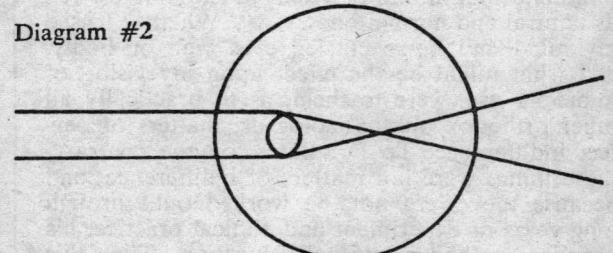

The myopic eye (nearsighted eye)
The light rays fall in front of the retina.

which the curvature of the cornea is abnormal so that light rays from the object regarded are diffused on the retina, and blurring occurs. Since what is wrong in all of these cases lies in the eyes, the correction for all of these conditions is the same—glasses.

Causes? I recall my own doctor's explanation when I got my first pair of glasses at age 12. It consisted essentially of the following from *Gifford's Textbook of Ophthalmology*[1]:

> The most important cause of axial myopia is heredity, in the sense of a hereditary tendency for the axial length of the eyes to reach abnormal proportions in the course of growth.

> Ever since ophthalmology became a science, its practitioners have been obsessively preoccupied with only one aspect of the total, complex process of seeing—the physiological. They have paid attention exclusively to eyes, not at all to the mind which makes use of the eyes to see with. I have been treated by men of the highest eminence in their profession; but never once did they so much as faintly hint that there might be a mental side to vision, or that there might be wrong ways of using the eyes and mind as well as right ways, unnatural and abnormal modes of visual functioning as well as natural and normal ones. . . . Whether I used my mind and be-spectacled eyes well or badly, and what might be the effect upon my vision of improper use, were to them, as to practically all other orthodox ophthalmologists, matters of perfect indifference. To Dr. Bates, on the contrary, these things were not matters of indifference; and because they were not, he worked out, through long years of experiment and clinical practice, his peculiar method of visual education. That this

[1] *Gifford's Textbook of Ophthalmology*. W. B. Saunders, Co., 1957, p. 113.

method was essentially sound, is proved by its efficacy.

—Aldous Huxley
The Art of Seeing,
Barbara Krohn and Associates, 1942, pp. x, xi.

The eye is the organ of vision, and resembles a photographer's camera in its construction. The iris is the diaphragm, with a pupillary opening in the center, which adjusts itself to the amount of light by dilating or contracting. Like the camera, the vitreous chamber is darkened inside by the pigmented layer of the choroid. The retina, or nervous layer, is the sensitive plate of the camera, and receives the impression or image of the object. The crystalline lens is so adjusted by the aid of the ciliary muscle as to bring the light to a focus on the retina. In order to accomplish its function successfully all the media of the eye must be transparent. These media are from before backwards the cornea, the aqueous humor, the crystalline lens, and the vitreous humor. Any haziness of one or more of these media will, of course, interfere with the visual function. The first essential, then, of perfect vision is an absolute transparency of all the media, and the second is an accurate focusing of the rays of light on the retina through the adjustment of the crystalline lens. These impressions when received upon the retina are gathered up and concentrated, as it were, in the optic nerve, through which they are carried to the brain. In short-sighted persons the eye-ball is too long, while in far-sighted persons the eye-ball is too short, and the focal point, therefore, falls behind the retina. In either case a blurred image is received upon the retina. In order to overcome this blurring, and thus correct the optical defect, the eye unconsciously makes an effort by which the ciliary muscle acts on the lens. This effort explains why eye-strain may cause pain and discomfort. An optical correction for the refractive error is found in spectacle lenses. . . .

—Francis Heed Adler, M.D.
Gifford's Textbook of Ophthalmology,
W.B. Saunders Co., 1957, p. 37.

I don't know whose heredity I was supposed to have. In my immediate family, my father was farsighted, my mother normal. My sister had myopia in one eye, my brother and other sister had normal vision, and I was myopic in both eyes. Grandparents on neither side wore glasses, and my aunts and uncles also all appeared to have normal vision up until their middle years, when some of them had to wear reading glasses, a condition quite different from mine. No doctor ever asked about the family's vision. I was told simply that my eyeballs had grown too long and that it "ran in the family." I guess someone back in the family line must have carried the "germs" of myopia, which I was singled out to catch.

Here is the cause for farsightedness, from the same source[2]:

> The principal cause of hyperopia (farsightedness) . . . is heredity.

Same cause, but different eyeball length. In hyperopia it is too short.

Astigmatism?

> In nearly all cases astigmatism is a congenital condition in which heredity is the only known factor. . . .[3]

Certainly vision has to do with the way we perceive things. And certainly it has to do with images or pictures that have form, color and light. Surely our eyes are the organs designed for this sort of perception. Yet, if you close your eyes and someone suggests that you imagine (notice how the word *image* is contained in the word *imagine*) a bright red paper kite flying against a

---

[2] *Ibid.*, pg. 110.
[3] *Ibid.*

blue sky, you would be able to *see* it—that is, you would form a picture inside your mind. When you sleep and dream, you also *see* things, and quite vividly. In both these instances, your eyes are not receiving any stimulus, yet you are *seeing*. Vision must therefore include something other than the eyes alone, or we would not be able to see in these ways. Granted, the eyes are no doubt necessary in order for *imaging* in this way to occur, but something else is functioning in the act of seeing and is essential to it. If this is so, then perhaps it is that "something else" that malfunctions in the case of poor vision, whether the affliction is nearsightedness, farsightedness, or whatever.

Dr. Bates proposed a theory of vision that included this other element. He proposed that it was the *mind* that completed the act of seeing an object, and that the mind had a lot more to do with proper seeing than had previously been acknowledged. Perhaps that was too obvious, because very few of Bates's peers thought much of his idea; or perhaps it was and is because so little was and is known of this mind of ours.

The mind is not something that can be cut up and analyzed in the way that an organ can, with tidy diagrams showing each part and its function.

The eye can be considered an optical instrument having a number of surfaces of different curvature and different refractive index through which the light rays have to pass. By far the largest portion of the refraction of rays of light is accomplished at the surface of the cornea, for here the rays enter from a medium, air, with an index refraction of 1.0 into a medium, the cornea, with an index refraction of 1.33. . . . After passing through the cornea, the rays emerge into the aqueous, which has practically the same index of refraction. They then strike a second medium of greater optical density, namely, the lens. Here further bending of the rays takes place, but much less than on the anterior surface of the cornea since the rays are moving from the aqueous, index of refraction 1.33, into the lens, index of refraction 1.42. As the rays emerge from the lens into the vitreous, they enter a medium of less density and are therefore slightly diverged. As a result of the bending of rays by all these surfaces, they come to a focus on the retina if the eye is normal and if the entering rays are parallel to the optic axis.[4]

The above description reflects our particular Western world view, which happens to be predominantly a mechanistic one—one that we tend to trust, however, as *factual*, *objective*, and an *accurate* description of reality. We pride ourselves on this. The mystery of seeing, the wonder of such a process, gets reduced in this view to the level of the internal combustion engine. A riddle such as how the rods and cones in the retina transmit messages to the optic nerve so that sight occurs gets shelved until a mechanical description can be found.

Bates, a scientist and empiricist himself, did not get into a poetry of vision, but, using scientific methods together with a fine intelligence, he did extend a description of vision into the less easily described "mind." (Note that he used the term *mind* and not *brain*.) I suggest that it was because his ideas, based on this nebulous "mind," countered the mechanistic leanings of Western science and medicine that his work was condemned and ignored in spite of the incredible results he achieved. Dr. Bates used intuition along with reason, asked more questions than he could answer with mechanical solutions that would please his peers. His thinking came much closer to Zen Buddhism than to a description of the internal combustion engine. Vision to

---

[4] Ibid., pg. 107.

him was a *process* that ended in the unexplained regions of the "mind." With such a theory, solutions for poor vision could no longer be found in glasses. A much more holistic approach had to be found. And Bates went looking for one.

CHAPTER 2
William H. Bates, Vision-ary

William H. Bates was an ophthalmologist with degrees from Cornell University and the College of Physicians and Surgeons in New York. He practiced at the Manhattan Eye and Ear Hospital, the New York Eye Infirmary, Bellevue Hospital, the Northwestern Dispensary, and Harlem Hospital. He did 40 years of his own research before he presented his findings to the American Medical Association. Yet in 1976, there was no mention of Dr. Bates or his work in any section of the card catalogue of the UCLA Medical School library. His findings were not only unrecognized and undocumented; they were buried as if they had never been formally presented. The medical profession does not need to burn books; it simply refuses to make public ideas that do not agree with the existing structure. Like so many alternatives to the medical monopoly, the Bates work went underground, kept alive by people who had experienced its results.

> **Journal Entry**
>
> *August 11, 1975*
>
> Started eye exercises a week-and-a-half ago. Whole insight into self. I am so closed, as if there really were a barrier between me and outside, even with sound, as with music I don't let in, or people, or all sorts of things. I am literally cut off visually; it amazes me how little I see. Even driving, I am like the mechanical woman. Anyway, it's an exciting, frustrating experience. I want to see *now*! Go to eye doctor this week. We'll see.

For years, like all eye doctors, Bates had put glasses on people. Gradually, however, he began to question this "solution." He wondered why it was assumed that the eye was the only organ of the body that apparently could not repair itself. This seemed most peculiar since the body had such highly developed systems of defense and repair in other, less critical, areas.

Because the proper functioning of the eye was central to the way an organism obtained external information essential to its well-being and survival, it did not seem likely that nature would neglect the eye in this way. Similarly, it did not make sense to him that the eye had not made the adjustment to civilized life—which still is one of the underlying assumptions for the prevalence of poor vision in the modern world.

Eons before there were any schools or printing presses, electric lights or moving pictures, the evolution of the eye was complete. In those days it served the needs of the human animal perfectly. Man was a hunter, a herdsman, a farmer, a fighter. He needed, we are told, mainly distant vision; and since the eye at rest is adjusted for distant vision, sight is supposed to have been ordinarily as passive as the perception of sound, requiring no muscular action whatever. Near vision, it is assumed, was the exception, necessitating a muscular adjustment of such duration that it was accomplished without placing any appreciable burden upon the mechanism of accommodation [the adjustment of the eye to different distances]. The fact that primitive woman was a seamstress, an embroiderer, a weaver, an artist of all sorts of fine and beautiful work, appears to have been generally forgotten. Yet women living under primitive conditions have just as good eyesight as men.[1]

Bates also wondered why a person developed vision problems after seeing perfectly in early childhood. Why did the eyeball elongate permanently as in myopia (nearsightedness) or flatten as in hyperopia (farsightedness) so that blurred vision at either the far or near point resulted? His concern led him to question the theory fundamental to the ophthalmological profession—the theory of accommodation first proposed by Helmholtz in the nineteenth century.

Accommodation refers to the eye's ability to change focus rapidly from the far to near point. As stated earlier, the eye at rest is adjusted to see objects in the distance; in order to see objects nearby, it must make some adjustment, just as a camera must be adjusted for near and distant objects. According to Helmholtz, it was the lens inside the eye that changed shape in order to project the image onto the retina, located at the back of the eye (see Diagram 3). But Dr. Bates, like other ophthalmologists, was aware of a significant number of people whose lenses had been totally removed as a result of a cataract operation, but whose eyes still possessed, to some degree, the ability to accommodate.

---

[1] Bates, William H., M.D., *Better Eyesight without Glasses*. Holt, Rinehart & Winston, 1978, pp. 9–10.

Diagram #3
Schematic Section of the Human Eye

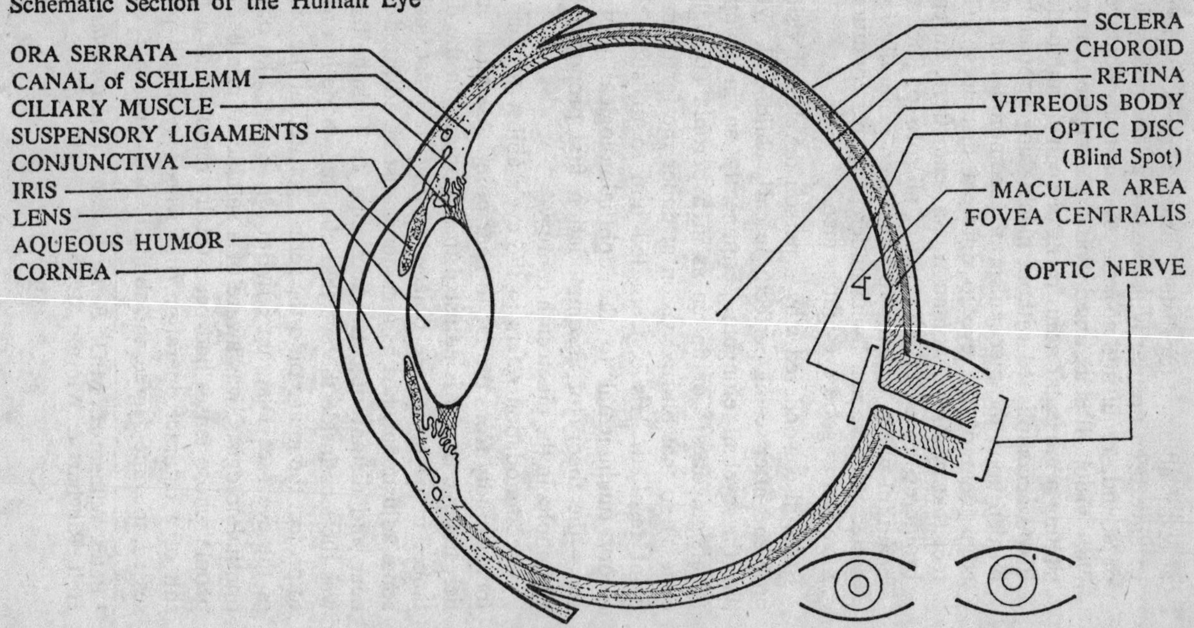

- ORA SERRATA
- CANAL of SCHLEMM
- CILIARY MUSCLE
- SUSPENSORY LIGAMENTS
- CONJUNCTIVA
- IRIS
- LENS
- AQUEOUS HUMOR
- CORNEA
- SCLERA
- CHOROID
- RETINA
- VITREOUS BODY
- OPTIC DISC (Blind Spot)
- MACULAR AREA
- FOVEA CENTRALIS
- OPTIC NERVE

It particularly bothered Dr. Bates to put glasses on young children. It was this and other questions and observations that led him to begin four years of experimentation using animals and fish as his subjects. He would remove the lens of an eye. The eye still showed an ability to accommodate. Then he would cut one or several of the muscles that surround the eye globe. The eye could not accommodate any longer. He would suture the muscle back together; the eye could accommodate once again.

> Examining thousands of pairs of eyes a year at the New York Eye and Ear Infirmary and other institutions, I observed many cases in which errors of refraction either recovered spontaneously or changed their form, and I was unable either to ignore them or to satisfy myself with the orthodox explanations, even where such explanations were available. It seemed to me that if a statement is a truth, it must always be a truth. There can be no exceptions. If errors of refraction are incurable, they should not recover, or change their form, spontaneously.
>
> —William H. Bates, M.D.,
> *Better Eyesight without Glasses,*
> Holt, Rinehart & Winston, 1978, p. 14.
>
> There are also people who regain their near vision after having lost it for ten, fifteen, or more years, and there are people who, while presbyopic for some objects, have perfect sight for others. Many dressmakers, for instance, can thread a needle with the naked eye . . . and yet they cannot read or write without glasses.
>
> So far as I am aware, no one but myself has ever observed the last-mentioned class of cases, but the others are known to every ophthalmologist of any experience. One hears of them at the meetings of ophthalmological societies, they are even

> reported in the medical journals; but such is the force of authority that when it comes to writing books they are either ignored or explained away, and most of the new treatises that come from the press repeat the old superstition that presbyopia is "a normal result of growing old." The dead hand of German science still oppresses our intellects and prevents us from crediting the plainest evidence of our senses. German ophthalmology is still sacred, and no facts are allowed to cast discredit upon it.
>
> —William H. Bates, M.D.
> *Better Eyesight without Glasses*, p. 31.

> Any community of people holds in common certain assumptions about reality. Our language itself is a set of common assumptions, shared for the convenience of easy discourse. "No one can run a mile in less than four minutes" was another. Each scientific community, of physicists, mathematicians, psychologists, or others, shares an additional set of implicit assumptions, called the *paradigm* by Thomas Kuhn. The paradigm is the shared conceptions of what is possible, the boundaries of acceptable inquiry, the limiting cases.
>
> The working of the scientific paradigm is similar to the working of an individual's assumptions about reality. Personal categories are by their nature conservative of effort. . . . Within science, a paradigm allows a similar stability of knowledge, again at the price of a certain insensitivity to new input. . . . But there is a danger here: parochialism. Just as the residents of a certain community may become smug about their town and consider it the "only" place in the world, so the scientist working under a successful paradigm may begin to lose sight of any possibilities beyond his own particular set of assumptions.
>
> —Robert E. Ornstein,
> *The Psychology of Consciousness*,
> Penguin Books, 1979, pp. 19–20, 22.

Dr. Bates also observed hundreds of his patients, using the retinoscope. His experiments and observations led him to the conclusion that it was not the lens but the extrinsic eye muscles that were principally responsible for accommodation. He theorized that these muscles *tensed* when a person strained to see, or as a result of general stress, and that the tension created a distortion of the eyeball, causing the retina to lock in a position either too far forward or too far back to permit the image entering the eye to fall directly upon it as nature intended. Thus, blurring occurred. According to his idea, the normal eye changed shape constantly as the person moved his attention from near to far and from object to object located at different distances. Tense eyes lost this flexibility; they locked for vision within a limited range.

With this discovery, Dr. Bates proposed the theory fundamental to all the Bates exercises—that it is tension in the mind that causes the muscles to contract, thus distorting the shape of the eyeball and causing poor vision. With this as his basis, he directed his attention to developing techniques that would relax the tension. Years of trial and error went into the development of these exercises. Bates had both successes and failures, but his successes far outnumbered his failures. He would make his patients throw their glasses away and have them practice the various techniques he developed. He helped people not only with the common visual problems, but also people with glaucoma, cataracts, detached retinas, and crossed eyes. He even helped blind people.

Margaret Corbett had no vision problem. But her husband's vision was poor and growing worse, and no one had been able to stop the deterioration. Mr. Corbett ended up at Dr. Bates's New York clinic and grad-

> The mind is the source of all . . . efforts from outside sources brought to bear upon the eye. Every thought of effort in the mind, of whatever sort, transmits a motor impulse to the eye, and every such impulse causes a deviation from the normal in the shape of the eyeball and lessens the sensitiveness of the center of sight.
>
> —William H. Bates, M.D.,
> *Better Eyesight without Glasses,* p. 47.
>
> Primarily, the strain to see is a strain of the mind, and, as in all cases in which there is a strain of the mind, there is a loss of mental control. Anatomically, the results of straining to see at a distance may be the same as those of regarding an object at the near-point without strain, but in one case the eye does what the mind desires and in the other it does not.
>
> These facts appear to explain . . . why vision declines as civilization advances. Under the conditions of civilized life, men's minds are under a continual strain.
>
> —William H. Bates, M.D.,
> *Better Eyesight without Glasses,* p. 40.

ually regained normal sight. His wife was amazed and grateful and became a Bates enthusiast. It was particularly distressing to her that all of Dr. Bates's work was being completely ignored by his medical peers. She studied the Bates techniques herself and returned to Los Angeles to establish a Bates school, where she trained teachers and helped hundreds of people to improve or completely regain their vision. Aldous Huxley, whose vision was failing to the point of total blindness, regained vision completely in one eye and was able to salvage the near-blindness of his weaker eye so that he could continue his life's work. Out of gratitude he wrote his marvelous book called *The Art of Seeing*.

The Bates movement reached its flowering in the late '30s and early '40s. During World War II, the United States government called upon Margaret Corbett's school to help develop perfect night vision in pilots assigned to fly night bombing missions. But in 1941, Margaret Corbett was accused of practicing optometry without a license. Although she was acquitted, the experience proved devastating for her. She became anxious about her work, fearing each new student to be a spy trying to catch her in statements that might be used against her.

She was not practicing optometry—the Bates method works at relaxing the *mind*, aims at freeing the eyes so that they will do what comes naturally to them. But the professionals apparently were jealous of her success. Bates teachers have been hauled into court from time to time. Not one has ever been convicted of the charges, but being arrested became one of the professional hazards of being a Bates teacher.

Margaret Corbett died in 1961. With her death, the Bates movement lost a lot of its impetus. Seven years later, the association of teachers dissolved itself. Today, there are perhaps three to four dozen Bates teachers left in the United States.

But the possibility of a Bates renaissance remains. Doctors today seem to be a little more receptive to the unorthodox alternatives that have sprung up all over the country in all areas of health and nutrition. Perhaps some of these men and women may reinvestigate the work that Dr. Bates did. In the meantime, the few Bates teachers left are still teaching, and people who want an alternative to glasses are still flocking to them. Dr. Bates is dead, still unrecognized for his work. But there are thousands of people who remember him and are grateful for what he did for them. He was a true scientist, a pioneer probing and questioning and bringing hope and relief to the world. Perhaps someday soon he will gain his rightful place in the annals of medicine.

> The visual area [of the brain] registers electrical stimuli received from the retina as meaningless patterns of light. The visual association zone decodes and makes sense of the impulses registered in the visual area, but it does not form an actual image from the impulses. There is no inner eyeball that "sees" a pictorial representation in the brain. This decoding process is a learned ability. People blind from birth whose sight is restored through surgery only perceive light. They have to learn to turn light patterns into meaningful images.
>
> —Mike Samuels, M.D., and Nancy Samuels,
> *Seeing with the Mind's Eye,*
> Random House, 1979, pp. 57–58.
>
> Errors of refraction, including presbyopia . . . are due not to an organic change in the shape of the eyeball or in the constitution of the lens, but in a functional derangement in the action of the muscles on the outside of the eyeball, and therefore can be eliminated.
>
> —William H. Bates, M.D.,
> *Better Eyesight without Glasses,* p. 15.

CHAPTER 3
Seeing and vision

For the sake of differentiation, *seeing* might be defined as the simple act of receiving, via the eyes, information that is then transmitted to the brain; *vision*, then, is the act of perception, of synthesis and understanding of that information. One of the earliest developments in the life of a fetus is the protrusion of the optic nerve from the brain; if fact, the optic nerve is an extension of the brain and opens, fanlike, to become the innermost sensitive lining of the eye, the retina. An infant only "sees"; "vision" develops over a period of time through the repetition of information, so that the information is then "recognized." At about three months of age, a baby seems to recognize its parents; this may be the child's first vision. Seeing, then, occurs in the eyes and brain. Vision occurs in the mind.

Until this century, when Dr. Bates began to probe the causes of defective vision, ophthalmologists concerned themselves solely with seeing, not vision. Most today continue to follow this path, although, based on the work of a Dr. A. M. Skeffington, who also challenged the conventionally held theories of ophthalmology, a new school of optometrics has gotten a foothold in vision training. Because of this concentration on seeing rather than vision, the science of ophthalmology has offered its patients virtually no hope for the improvement of eyesight other than through lenses. Once the distinction between seeing and vision is made, however, a door opens into new possibilities.

To a large extent, seeing can be explained through a description of the eye structure itself. Starting from the brain and moving forward to the surface of the eye, we have first the optic nerve, which, as already stated, is an extension of the brain itself. It carries the visual information, via nerve impulses, to the visual centers of the brain, where interpretation, i.e. vision, then occurs. The retina is the receiving end of the optic nerve; it is a delicate lining that forms the backmost inner part of the eyeball. The retina is often compared to the film inside a camera, where the pictures—and in the eye, the images—are registered.

The retina is composed of ten layers. The ninth, next to the innermost, is the most important, as it contains the rods and cones—specialized nerve ends that do the job of seeing. Near the center of the retina, there is a small yellowish area called the macula lutea, where sight is the sharpest. It is also here where the greatest number of cones are concentrated. In the center of the macula lutea is a small pit, called the fovea centralis, where an even more sensitive group of cones are located. The rods are situated toward the outer edges of the retina. The cones are presumed to distinguish colors and are the cells that aid our daylight vision; the rods aid our night vision and peripheral vision.

In the normal, relaxed eye, the image of the object viewed falls upon the macula area, so that a clear, sharp picture is registered and transmitted to the brain. In the subnormal eye, the image falls either in front of, behind, or to one side of the macula; thus, only a blurred image can be sent for interpretation. In myopia, the eyeball is abnormally elongated, causing the image to fall in front of the macula. In hyperopia, the eyeball is too short, so that the image theoretically falls behind the macula.

The retina is coated with a chemical called rhodopsin, or visual purple. Scientists do not agree about how the visual purple functions in the act of seeing, because none of it is present in the macula itself. It seems to be used, however, in much the same way a chemical wash is used in developing film—it helps to "develop" the image. But where film developers are used up in the process of development, the visual purple is immediately replaced, enabling the eye to receive images continuously without interruption.

Although blood vessels are plentiful in the eye, none are located in the macular area. And though there are rods and cones intermixed all through the retina, there are only a few rods in the macula and none in the fovea. The cones decrease in number toward the outer portions of the retina, while the number of rods increases. It is because of the location of the rods that we see an object at night by looking a bit to one side of the object so that the image falls, not centrally on the now insensitive cones, but outside the macular area, where the rods can perceive in the dim light. It is also because of these rods that we have peripheral vision.

Try this experiment: choose an object directly in front of you, and focus your attention on it. You will be viewing the object with macular, or central vision. Now hold up your hands on either side of your head, palms forward, so you are just aware of something out at the sides. Wiggle your fingers to catch your peripheral sight. You will recognize that some object is on either side of your head, but until you move your hands further forward, you will not perceive the objects as your hands. As you move your hands further and further forward toward your center of sight, you begin to see them for what they are.

The retina is the most delicate and important part of the eye and is generously protected by two outer coatings that encase it. It is even further protected by the vitreous fluid that fills the hollow of the eye.

The outer covering, the sclera, which completely encircles the globe of the eye except where it is pierced by the optic nerve, is a tough opaque covering composed of numerous layers so that the eye is well-protected even if one layer is bruised or scratched. In the front of the eyeball, the sclera forms the white of the eye and becomes transparent like the crystal of a watch. This frontal area is called the cornea. The cornea has five layers, one of which is a tough sheath that protects the eye from injury. Further protection is afforded by the eyelid, which often closes against a foreign object before we even have time to think about doing the action consciously. The eyelid also helps to wash the cornea with the salty, antibacterial solution produced by the tear glands.

Under the multilayers of the sclera is another coating, the choroid lining. This layer is dark and allows no light to pass through it so that the interior of the eyeball remains dark, except where light enters through the pupil. The choroid contains a concentration of blood vessels that provide the nutrients essential to the retina, as well as the veins that carry away waste. It too is multilayered, and it contains one thin, shell-like layer that further protects the retinal tissues that lie just within the choroid, attached to it for nourishment.

The choroid reaches two-thirds of the way around the eye globe toward the front, where it becomes the ciliary body, the function of which is still in dispute. The iris sits in front of the ciliary; it, the choroid, and ciliary body are of the same tunic. The iris is the colored part of the eye, which opens and closes, regulating the amount of light that enters the eye through its opening, the pupil. The iris opens wide in dim light, closes to almost a pinpoint in bright light. The lens, which contains a series of layers of transparent tissue, floats behind the iris in a small capsule of fluid. Light entering the eye through the pupil passes through the lens, whereby it is directed back to the retina.

The aqueous, a clear, watery fluid, fills the spaces beneath the cornea, around the iris and lens, and is responsible for holding these parts in position and shape. Another, more viscous fluid, called the vitreous, fills the hollow inside the eye, maintaining the contours of the eyeball.

The eyeball is surrounded by three pairs of muscles attached to the outside wall of the sclera. (See Diagram 4) Two of these pairs, called the recti muscles, attach near the cornea and reach back to the bony structure at the back of the eyeball. One pair attaches to the top and bottom of the eye; the other pair attaches to either side. The third pair, called the obliques, encircle the eye; one muscle attaches to the under portion, the other to the upper portion.

These muscles function in two ways. On the one hand, they are striated muscles, thus voluntary. This means we can consciously control them, and we do, to move our eyes up, down, and sideways. But where these muscles attach to the sclera, they are smooth. Smooth muscles are controlled by the involuntary nervous system, which means we cannot consciously control them. It is these smooth segments of the muscles that Dr. Bates discovered operate to elongate or flatten the eyeball in order to see near and far. Because light rays from a nearby object enter the eye at a different angle than light rays from a far object do, to see with macular vision, the retina must be moved back. The external muscles accomplish this by compressing the eye so that it elongates for near vision. For distant objects,

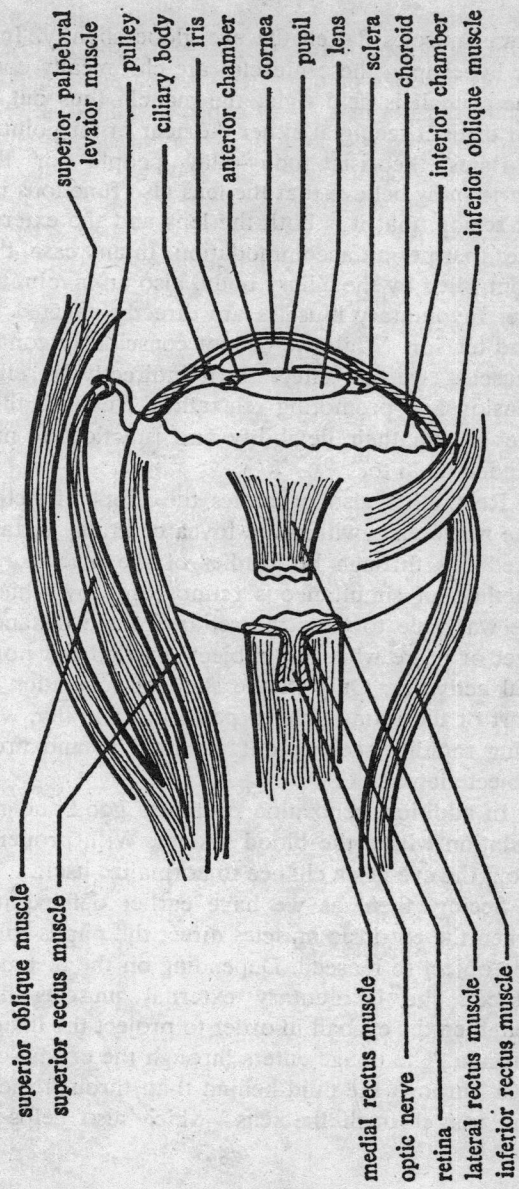

Diagram #4
Structure & Muscles of the Eye

these muscles flatten the eye globe slightly. In myopia or hyperopia, these muscles are chronically contracted; the eyeball is held rigid, the macula thus out of reach for distinct seeing at either the near or far point.

Bates theorists today—lay people for the most part—now believe that the lens also functions in the act of seeing, that it is both the lens and the external muscles that permit accommodation. In any case, the lens is controlled by the ciliary body, also an involuntary muscle. Involuntary muscles are directly affected by stress and tension. While we cannot consciously control these muscles, we can affect them indirectly by eliminating tension and promoting relaxation. Relaxed, these muscles regain their flexibility and function as nature intended them to.

Relaxation also promotes the proper functioning of the nerve ends within the fovea centralis. Bates discovered this through his studies of the macula, using his method of simultaneous retinoscopy, by which means he was able to view the retina from a distance of six feet or more while his subjects carried out normal visual activities. Only in the state of relaxation was this part of the retina able to perform naturally, with lightning rapidity seeking out the light in and around the object viewed.

In addition, relaxation promotes good and rapid circulation within the blood system. With proper circulation, the eye has a chance to normalize itself.

Seeing, then, as we have earlier defined it, occurs when the extrinsic muscles direct the pupils to focus on the object to be seen. Depending on the distance of the object, the involuntary external muscles flatten or lengthen the eyeball in order to project the image on the macula. The image enters through the crystal-clear cornea, through the fluid behind that, through the pupil of the iris, through the lens—which also helps to focus and concentrate the light—through the thicker vitreous fluid back to the cones and rods located in the retina. The light from the object frees the cones of the fovea into activity in which they seek out light all around and in the object viewed, to form an image. This picture is then transmitted via the optic nerve to the visual centers of the brain. There is no actual "image" in the brain; the "image" is sent by nerve impulses, a kind of code that the brain can interpret. In the visual centers, the mind completes the process of interpretation, making "sense" out of the information, relating it to its past experience and to the imagination, by which the picture is truly perceived. Thus, vision occurs. (See Diagram 5.)

That vision is a mental process can be clearly understood by examining a few details. For example, the image that occurs on the retina is reversed, i.e., is upside down. Yet the mind sees it right side up. Even when an object is viewed upside down, the mind will interpret correctly.

Furthermore, vision occurs most easily and rapidly when we view objects that are familiar to us. When a Westerner looks at any sequence of the letters of the alphabet with which he is familiar, he can identify the words, and the idea behind the words, with ease and speed. Presented with a new language, particularly when first learning a language that uses a different alphabet, such as Arabic or Chinese, he will miss important details in the formation of those symbols, details the native speaker would not miss. Even with careful observation, the learner will have difficulty "seeing" the strange signs. A country dweller, used to noticing minute changes in his landscape, will notice details, obvious to him, that a city dweller will not "see" unless specifically pointed out to him.

Seeing takes in everything, but vision is conditioned by our past experience, by that store that goes to make

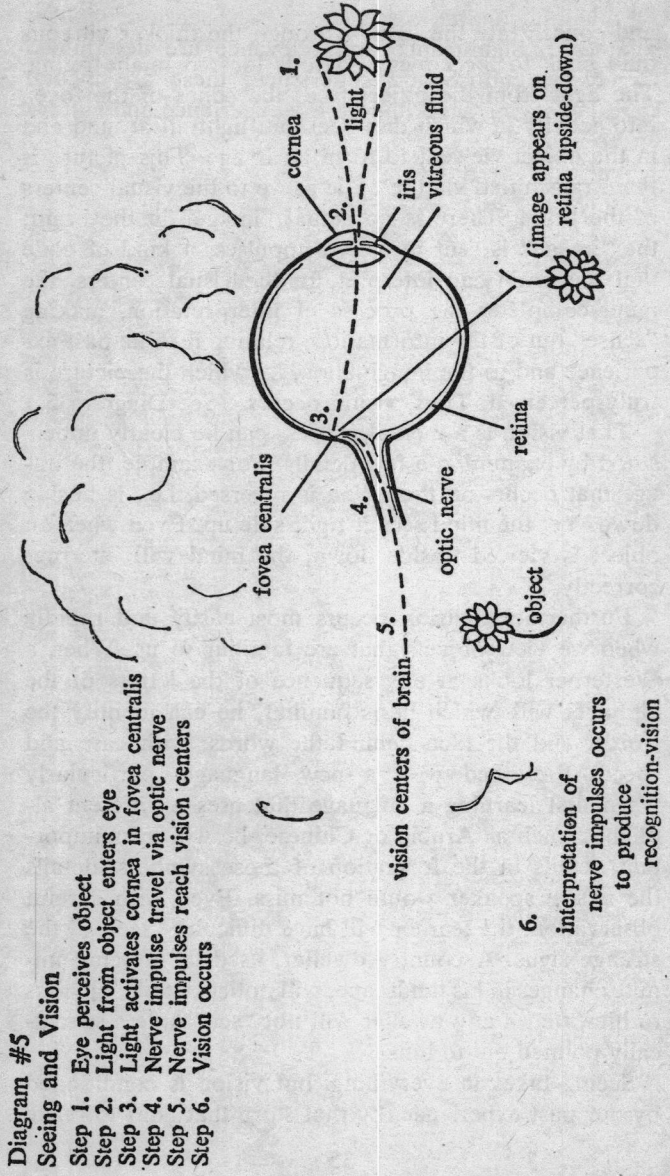

Diagram #5
Seeing and Vision

Step 1. Eye perceives object
Step 2. Light from object enters eye
Step 3. Light activates cornea in fovea centralis
Step 4. Nerve impulse travel via optic nerve
Step 5. Nerve impulses reach vision centers
Step 6. Vision occurs

up our imagination, our memory, our sense of what is significant. Significance and relevance are determined largely by culture and experience; these are mental states, changing according to the experience and culture of the individual.

An infant senses a mass of vague shapes—*sensa* as Huxley calls them. These *sensa* have no meaning or significance to him; in fact, we cannot even be sure that an infant can clearly delineate one object from another at first, just as a nonreader of Arabic cannot recognize where one word begins and ends out of the string of symbols on a page. But by observing any newborn during its first year of life, we notice how he gradually begins to discriminate, deriving pleasure or pain from the objects that now impinge on his consciousness.

When a person has a normal pair of eyes and brain, seeing is a function of simply being alive; vision develops out of accumulated experiences and a memory capable of retaining a store of past experience. In adults that store is readily available so that sensing and perceiving occur simultaneously. Under the influence of alcohol or a drug, a person can experience a somewhat disconnected world in which objects seem to have little or no relevance, in which there seems to be no "sense," no connection between one object and another. The person *sees* objects, but has no perception of them because of the distortion of the mind by the drug.

Vision is, of course, impossible without seeing. The data must be received for the mind to have anything to interpret from outside its own memory and imagination. And seeing must have occurred at some point in order for vision to develop. People born blind have no inner images; people who later become blind through injury or disease continue to have inner vision through their stored memories. The two processes are truly one, and the one (eyes or mind) affects the other. But where the emphasis in the past has always been on the eyes, now, with an understanding of the whole visual process, of what vision really is, it should be clear that your eyes are only a part of the process.

The Bates Method works with vision, not seeing, and with the strain that causes defective vision. When strain is eliminated, the defects of the eye correct themselves. Conventional ophthalmologists work the other way around. They believe that the eye defect causes the strain and thus treat the defect, permitting the strain to continue. In other words, they treat the symptoms, not the cause. Because the basis of the Bates Method is relaxation, and because stress and tension are the sources of so many other physical and mental problems, other health benefits accrue as the exercises are practiced and stress is eliminated.

The mind can think only one thing at a time. It does this so rapidly, however, that it appears to be dealing with numerous things simultaneously. The mind likewise cannot cling tediously to one detail, but moves around it, examining, interpreting, appreciating, always on the move. That the mind centralizes on one thing continuously, but ever moving, is important also in pain control. If you can remove your consciousness from your perception of pain to another idea or event, you will stop perceiving pain so acutely, sometimes even entirely.

The eye functions very similarly to the mind. The fovea "sees" only a pinpoint of any object clearly at any one time, but it moves so rapidly all over and around the object that it seems that we see the whole object at once. This one-pointedness combined with rapid and constant movement is the essence of consciousness.

The Bates techniques use this understanding to educate the eye/mind both to centralize and to move in order to achieve perfect vision. There is an apparent paradox, however. Neither centralization nor the lightninglike natural movement of eye and mind can be consciously sought, nor can they be achieved by any effort whatsoever. They come only as a result of relaxation. Relaxation can be consciously achieved. This is the essence of the Bates work.

CHAPTER 4
In-sight: Mind and vision

Close your eyes. Imagine a telephone pole two blocks away. How does it appear? Are its edges crisp and clear? How many wires attach to it? How many footholds are there?

Now imagine your own hand held a few inches in front of your nose. Is it clear or blurred? Or can you visualize it at all? Typically, people with low visual acuity have trouble visualizing in their minds. Their inner images are vague, fleeting or, when achieved, blurred and accompanied by a feeling of strain. The inner vision is usually as bad or worse than the outer vision. The nearsighted person has the greatest difficulty imagining objects farther away than his or her myopic circle; the farsighted person experiences his/her greatest difficulty with objects nearby.

What is of interest here is this inner vision, the ability or inability to see internally. Many people, with or without normal vision, and most adults, tend to verbal-

> Seeing, as we usually speak of it, involves much more than exciting the cells of the retina. It involves more than the eye, it involves the mind. . . . The better people train their minds to perceive external images, the easier it becomes for them to imagine internal images as well. . . . People who see blindly will find it difficult to picture visual images in their mind.
>
> —Mike Samuels, M.D., and Nancy Samuels, *Seeing with the Mind's Eye*, p. 114.
>
> **Journal Entry**
>
> *September 5, 1975*
> I realized today more fully that my myopia is a psychological condition—that I must release myself from whatever deep anxiety I have to *see* without letting something else take over symptomatically. An opening, a vulnerability, releasing the conscious mind from its total control. Felt panic when I actually saw clearly today. Such energy.

ize their thoughts rather than create images; thus their overall inner visual ability to "see" things may not be as quick as that of people who naturally "image" things—e.g., children, and people of cultures that do not place so much emphasis on the word, or reading and writing, as we in the West do. *People with normal vision, however, will always visualize things clearly.*

If you see in a blurred fashion at either the near or far point, you will probably visualize in the same way. If you see clearly, you will visualize clearly. Bates discovered, however, that the converse is also true. When you develop your inner vision, you will improve your external vision. The eyes follow the mind. Bates also observed that when a person clearly imagined an object in the distance, his closed eyes adjusted to that distance; and when he imagined an object nearby, his eyes made that adjustment as well.

I have personally experienced this coordination of eye and mind in my own vision work, and have observed it in many students. One student, a man in his late forties, who was just beginning to become presbyopic, was perfectly able to imagine his hand held three inches in front of his face, but could not imagine print, letters, or numbers. When questioned, he remarked that, indeed, the only difficulty he was as yet experiencing was with reading; he could still see all other objects up close. He also noticed that his difficulties were less in the morning, increasing in severity as his busy day progressed. He expressed the typical cultural notions that middle age was a time when one should *expect* to see the beginnings of physical deterioration (see Chapter 4); in short, he expected his reading vision to fail.

> Wilder Penfield, among others, has demonstrated that the experience of vision can also be evoked by electrical stimulation of the central nervous system. Penfield performed brain surgery on patients with epilepsy and, as part of this procedure, electrically stimulated various areas of the brain; his patients often reported conscious experiences without any other input at all. For instance, many surgeons have found that electrical stimulation of the occipital cortex usually leads to the experience of vision. We can understand, then, that seeing is a process which takes place not *in* our eyes, but rather *with the help* of our eyes. It is a process that is constructed in the brain, one largely determined by the category and output systems of the brain.
> —Robert E. Ornstein,
> *The Psychology of Consciousness,* p. 60.

A nearsighted student, a woman in her early twenties, could not visualize a ball being tossed to another student standing about six feet in front of her. Or, rather, she could imagine the ball, but noted that it was "very blurry." I asked her to imagine the ball being tossed on a TV screen that was a few inches in front of her. No matter how "far" the ball was thrown on the TV screen, she could see it clearly now. Since she was "close," distance was no longer significant to her. Now, anyone can argue for the reality of distance when one's eyes are open, but what is distance in the imagination? Is it not simply an illusion? With the help of the imagined TV screen, this woman could "see" any distance; without it, she could not imagine clearly any object beyond a couple of feet. Yet this same young woman had dreams in which she visualized clearly all kinds of objects and people at all distances. Why?

It has been found that mental images have many of the same physical components as open-eyed perceptions. For example, researchers have found correlations between a person's eye movements and the moment he was dreaming of climbing stairs. In another study, it was found that people scanning their eidetic (i.e., memory) images moved their eyes just as if they were still viewing the external picture. The American physiologist Neisser has said that "visual images are apparently produced by the same integrative processes that make ordinary perception possible. . . . Visual memory differs from perception because it is based principally on stored, rather than on current information, but it involves the same kind of synthesis."

—Mike Samuels, M.D., and Nancy Samuels, *Seeing with the Mind's Eye*, p. 57.

> An extremely important purpose, indeed a central feature, of the new visual training is the reduction or elimination of stress. . . . The new school holds that defective vision is by definition stressful vision. . . .
>
> In one test, Dr. Amiel Francke asks the patient to begin multiplying in his head two times two times two times two—to infinity. . . . It is thus possible, in the space of a minute or so, to observe all of the possible variations in reflex as the patient goes from relaxed calculation into a stress response, which is a constriction of the visual system. If the stress is sustained, it leads in almost every case to semi-permanent visual distortions, chief among which is nearsightedness [myopia]. . . .
>
> —Ann and Townsend Hoopes,
> *Eye Power,* Alfred A. Knopf, 1979, pp. 68, 69, 74.

According to the science of ophthalmology, the causes of all of our visual defects are physiological: the trouble lies in the eyes. Thus the "cures" or solutions to the various problems are physical: glasses, medicines, surgery, etc. What causes the eyes to change from normal to abnormal is unclear; generally the explanation given is that these changes are genetic, or the result of too rapid growth, aging, or whatever.

Because Bates suggested that the mind might be the responsible agent, he had to go beyond such responses. He proposed that it was tension or strain in the *mind* that caused many visual difficulties, including myopia, hyperopia, astigmatism, glaucoma, and cataracts. The strain, he believed, was a *strain to see*.

Any doctor will tell you that tension results in tight muscles, and that tight muscles result in reduced physiological functioning. In any physical endeavor, we are at our best when we are relaxed. Furthermore, muscles that remain tense for an extended period of time create discomfort, pain, disease, or malfunction.

The strain to see creates tension in the muscles that surround the eye globe. Depending upon how intense the strain is, and for which distance, and/or kinds of objects, the eye muscles tighten, distorting the shape of the eyeball. An occasional strain will result in moments, perhaps unnoticed, of poor vision; continuous strain will result in a chronic condition of visual malfunction.

> Tension prohibits muscular relaxation. A muscle must relax. Relaxing is part of its function. If a muscle fails to relax, it stays tight. It loses its stretch, its suppleness, its give. Over a period of time, it becomes permanently shortened. When this happens, the muscle loses most of its ability to release tension. If you have tense and shortened muscles, you are susceptible to all sorts of "tension syndrome"—back pain, stiff neck, or headache—because your muscles never have the chance to let go or relax, and neither do you.
>
> —Hans Kraus, M.D.,
> *Backache, Stress, and Tension,*
> Pocket Books, 1972, p. 61.

Our inner vision is perhaps the accumulation of years of visual perception, the sum, so to speak, of memory. But it is also greater than that sum in its ability to create new forms, to invent visually. The importance of our inner vision here is that it illustrates the role the mind plays in seeing. If eyes were the only source of poor vision, why would this inner vision deteriorate as well? And if eyes are not the only source, then what *is* the cause of poor vision? Vision defects, like myopia, astigmatism, and hyperopia, usually *develop*—which means that the sufferer often had perfect vision for years. Where does it all begin?

In the introduction, I told of my own early experience with poor vision. When my own child, at about the same age, began to complain of difficulty seeing, I had her eyes checked. They were, fortunately, normal. But beyond seeing a doctor, both before and after the examination I frequently checked on her ability to see in the distance. I would ask her to read signs or numbers in the distance, doing this in such a way that she did not realize that she was being tested. What struck me then was the memory of my own parents' reaction to my first complaints about difficulty seeing: they had simply ignored them. Or so I thought. But being parents, they no doubt did what I had done: occasionally, and casually, checked my vision to find that I could see in the distance just fine. Like my own presbyopic student, my early myopia was very probably selective at first, limited to my fifth-grade classroom. My parents rightfully did not put me in glasses when I first asked for them; for most objects I was not yet myopic. Is it possible that most visual defects are initially selective (excepting, of course, those conditions caused by physical malfunction, disease, or injury)? If myopia is at first limited to certain situations, if a middle-aged person cannot read print 12 inches in front of him, but can thread a needle or otherwise see small objects at the same or less distance, what does all this imply?

Journal Entry,

June, 1976

I know my physical vision is deeply connected to my inner vision—I can tell by the degree of real panic I discover when I flash (i.e., see) clearly for a moment. *It is frightening to see.*

Journal Entry,
December 5, 1976

I flashed for the first time last night *at* night and in artificial lighting. Suddenly I saw A's painting across the room, almost sharp and clear. It was a real thrill. My glasses are too strong for me now, and I usually simply forget that I even need glasses. The blur has become my element, and I've gotten accustomed to it—my reality for the time being. But at least it's *true*, not overcome by false means—lenses—and it is *temporary*.

A large percentage of myopes develop their myopia between the ages of eight and ten. Dr. Bates suggested that this does not result from poor lighting, nor from the use of the eyes for close work, as has often been supposed, but to the constant *unfamiliarity* of material that schoolchildren are exposed to. When faced with familiar objects, the eye/mind complex easily takes in what appears before it—the brain identifies the object with ease, consequently with relaxation. But when presented with an unfamiliar object, the brain must search for suitable comparisons, must make an *effort* to identify the object.

In short, not only is the whole process of education a constant flow of unfamiliar objects and concepts, but the weight of personal failure that accompanies the educational process can make it a terrible burden for some children. The addition of this component may turn the brain's *effort* to identify unfamiliar material into chronic *strain*. ("Do you see?" the teacher asks, using *see* to mean *understand*. The subconscious is notoriously literal: *I do not see*, taken literally to mean the act of seeing, thus becomes the internal message.) To offset vision disorders brought on by schoolwork, Bates suggested having a Snellen eye chart conspicuously in view in all classrooms as a kind of visual anchor for students to go back to. The teachers were to use the chart several times during the day so that children could rest their eyes by regarding something thoroughly familiar. It was extremely successful for the time it was in use; in schools that correctly and consistently used this technique, the incidence of vision defects dropped off noticeably.

> To repeat a very important principle: you cannot see anything with perfect sight unless you have seen it before. When the eye looks at an unfamiliar object it always strains more or less to see that object, and an error of refraction is always produced. When children look at unfamiliar writings or figures on the blackboard, distant maps, diagrams, or pictures, the retinoscope always shows that they are myopic, though their vision may be absolutely normal under other circumstances. The same thing happens when adults look at unfamiliar distant objects. When the eye regards a familiar object, however, the effect is quite different. Not only can it be regarded without strain, but the strain of looking at unfamiliar objects later is lessened.
>
> —William H. Bates, M.D.,
> *Better Eyesight without Glasses,* p. 151.

Because the strain is attached only to the schoolwork, the eyes and mind may at first block vision only in the classroom. In the case of the farsighted child, the vision is blocked for reading. For such children it is the reading itself that becomes too much for the child, and he or she "withdraws" his near vision from print, retaining, however, good distance vision. In middle-age sight, unfamiliarity of material obviously cannot be the cause.

But what of our cultural expectations? How many people over 35 believe they will live fully, with great energy and unimpaired physical and mental funtioning, up until their seventies and eighties? Most people would consider such an optimistic attitude sheer Pollyannaism. We are conditioned to believe in our gradual decline; we fully *expect* to lose sexual vigor, vision, hearing, muscle tone—in fact all of our health and energy to a greater or lesser degree. Furthermore, we expect to see evidence of these losses in our forties and fifties. Do these expectations become self-fulfilling prophecies?

Journal Entry

August 7, 1976

Janet gave me an excellent lesson a few minutes ago. At the end, she spoke of how things just come into one, how one experiences a sensation almost of falling; one is abandoned to the world, letting it enter. I experienced it a moment, felt that incredible sensation of being *with* the tree I was looking at, not resisting it, or going out to meet it. She left then, and I began to cry. I am 37 years old, learning to see, not only with my eyes but with my being and my whole body. Learning after all these years of a dim, blurred world to be as I was born to be. . . . My crying, not hard or overwhelming, just there, a little, and needing to come out, was at the sense of how incredibly wasteful it is to live our lives so tight, so pulled in, how unnecessary our pain and suffering are, how lost to us so much beauty is—how *stupid* to bind our spirits so, as the Chinese used to bind their women's feet. All tied up and hard little bundles of fear. And of what? Indeed, what? The green leaves, the touch of wind or another person?

> Afraid to *feel* our bodies, to *be* what we are born to be? As if we could live only within the brain, as if the brain were not connected to these marvelous feeling, wanting bodies. Denying always—wishing to be separate spirits with all the ideals we give to the spiritual world, stealing from it the lovely sensations of physicality. . . . Real power for me is in the totality a person sends forth, how their mind, spirit, and body work together. Few are like that, but that's where I want to go, and it's body first, the first step I have to take. It begins with my eyes.

To recapitulate: Bates theorized that, for whatever reasons, the mind begins to strain to see; this strain causes tension in the muscles surrounding the eyeball, in turn causing the eyeball to distort in various ways. If the strain is unrelieved, the muscles remain tense, and the distortion worsens and/or becomes "permanent." Thus myopia, hyperopia, astigmatism, etc. are formed. Putting glasses on a person to "correct" the defect does not get at the cause; in fact, glasses usually worsen the condition. With Bates's explanation it is not so hard to understand how visual defects might at first be selective, disappearing in more relaxed circumstances, only to become fixed as the strain goes unrelieved.

It also becomes evident that the visual defect that results from the strain is a reaction that "saves" the viewer, or provides an "escape" from a stressful situation. If the viewer cannot *see* the object—be it print on the page or words on a chalkboard, he or she certainly cannot be expected to provide an appropriate response.

Of course the reaction need not stem necessarily or only from a school situation; it might result from any trauma or stressful event. Basically the viewer does not want to see something, or believes he cannot see (in the sense of understand); therefore he does not. Gradually the poor vision and the mental attitudes that reinforce poor vision become habits.

> That glasses must injure the eye is evident from the facts given in the preceding chapter. One cannot see through them unless one produces the degree of refractive errors which they are designed to correct. But refractive errors, in the eye which is left to itself, are never constant. If one secures good vision by the aid of concave, convex, or astigmatic lenses, therefore, it means that one is maintaining constantly a degree of refractive error which otherwise would not be maintained constantly. It is only to be expected that this should make the condition worse, and it is a matter of common experience that it does.
>
> —William H. Bates, M.D.,
> *Better Eyesight without Glasses*, p. 31.

One of these habits is the tendency to *stare*. All of life is movement; consciousness is movement; a lack of movement results in stagnation or death. Staring is essentially nonmovement, a visual clinging that results in the loss of visual consciousness of one's surroundings. Objects in the distance blur out for the myope; print disappears for the hyperope. The myope, particularly, walks around in a visual fog; even with glasses or lenses on, the myope is unusually unaware of his surroundings. For many hours of the day, he is functionally blind to the world around him.

Several other difficulties result from the inner strain to see: we become light-sensitive, avoiding the natural sunlight with dark glasses; we lose our night vision to a greater or lesser degree; and of course we lose the inner ability to visualize, becoming more and more dependent upon verbal and abstract modes of thinking and perceiving. Glasses do not alleviate any of these conditions.

The Bates techniques were developed to eliminate both the cause of poor vision and its principal effects. Thus, most of the exercises involve relaxation; all of them are done only after relaxation is achieved. And all of the exercises aim to reeducate the person to get movement back into his vision. Other exercises involve getting used to the natural sunlight, getting the two eyes to work together, and getting the mind to focus, to become visually alert once again. The process takes time; habits are often difficult to break. But everyone can improve his or her vision to some degree; with patience and practice, many can improve it back to the perfect vision they once had.

Journal Entry

August 25, 1976

Back from ophthalmologist. One year ago, I was 3.75 diopoters, saw 10/400 (this after a few weeks of Bates work when prescription was already too strong). In July (six weeks ago) I was 3.5 D., an improvement of ¼ diopoters. Today he gave me a 20/40 correction of 2 D, said I improved a ½ D in 6 weeks—looks to me like one full D, as I'm now closer to 2.5. When I see clearly with these new lenses (which have no astigmatism correction), I will be seeing 20/60. Quite an improvement.

CHAPTER 5
Seeing is believing

The French philosopher, Descartes, said, "I think, therefore I am." A contemporary might say, "I am what I think I am." One takes care of existence; the other takes care of identity. Both are ways of saying that mind creates being. To what extent this occurs can be seen more and more in the fields of physics, medicine, psychology, and the arts.

So much of Western thought has sprung out of the principles of dualism and separation: we are used to thinking of our bodies and minds as separate, discrete parts; science and religion have both taught us that; society constantly underscores it. The "new" learning, no doubt absorbed from Eastern religion and philosophy, suggests that body, mind and spirit are one and cannot be treated separately without doing harm.

> Bob Gilley, a 40-year-old executive with cancer, worked with Dr. Simonton using visualization. Before seeing Dr. Simonton, Gilley's survival was estimated at 30 percent. Of his work with visualization, Gilley has said, "I'd begin to visualize my cancer—as I saw it in my mind's eye. I'd make a game of it. The cancer would be a snake, a wolverine or some vicious animal. The cure, white husky dogs by the millions. It would be a confrontation of good and evil. I'd envision the dogs

> grabbing the cancer and shaking it, ripping it to shreds. The forces of good would win. The cancer would shrink . . . and then disappear. . . ." Gilley did this three times a day for 10- to 15-minute intervals. After six weeks of meditation, an examination revealed his tumor had shrunk by 75 percent. After two months Gilley had a cancer scan. There was no trace of the disease left in his body.
>
> —Mike Samuels, M.D., and Nancy Samuels, *Seeing with the Mind's Eye*, p. 227.

Dr. Carl Simonton, a radiologist who specializes in the treatment of cancer, has demonstrated how the mind and visualization techniques can shrink or eliminate deadly cancers. When patients cooperated by visualizing their cancers being attacked by "good" forces, the cancers were visibly reduced, and, in some cases, completely eliminated. Since Simonton works exclusively with terminal cancer patients, his work is most significant. And while he continues to use the traditional therapies, it is the mind, the use of visualization, that turns the tide. The traditional therapies alone had not worked, which is why his patients were terminal to begin with.

But it is not as if we have a tyrannical mind that runs the show alone. Communication between body and mind goes both ways; the body can talk back, can influence the mind. In their book, *Listening to the Body*, Dr. Jean Houston and Robert Masters show that we can alter our inner attitudes (our minds) by altering our bodies. They demonstrate how the body is a direct reflection of how we feel and think about ourselves. A particular posture, for example, accompanies a person's inner attitude toward himself. By making the person aware of the posture and getting him or her to change it, the mind will follow suit, changing the attitude, the self-image, that caused the posture. In some cases, it may be easier for a person to change his or her body posture than to consciously change the inner climate. A person with a negative self-image, for example, usually finds it very difficult to change that attitude merely by his own or outsiders' suggestions that he is better than he thinks he is. Such people can be helped more readily by Houston and Masters's more physical approach.

In the world of particle physics, the mind of the observer always changes the behavior of what is observed. In other words, if you are watching something, it will behave differently than when it is not watched. Such a discovery calls into question the "cold facts" of science, indeed the whole scientific method, which presupposes an "objective" universe that can be "objectively" verified and observed.

Contemporary painting, with its distortions and abstractions of objects, landscapes, and the human body, clearly reveals the mind at work creating new realities and forms and enlightening us to new ways of viewing existing forms. The reality portrayed in contemporary art is not the same as the one projected by artists prior to the twentieth century. A viewer might feel mystified by a contemporary painting, but if he simply allows himself to *see*, without looking for the old, he can usually sense the artist's intention and the underlying emotion.

By comparison to these recent observations and discoveries, Dr. Bates's theory—that the mind affects the eyes, that in the vast majority of cases *it* is responsible for poor vision—becomes less difficult to accept. Yet contemporary ophthalmologists still ridicule the idea. Even the "new" optometry, which accepts the notion that vision *can* be improved, and which at least acknowledges the mind as a component in the act of seeing, lacks the basic assumption that the mind *causes* poor vision.

> The new schools training optometrists agree . . . that the visual system embraces the eyes and the brain. They believe it is the "lead system" . . . the seat of command, the master coordinator for the whole body/mind system, receiving and synthesizing all the information supplied to it, integrating interpretation, ordering particular limb and body movements, and organizing intellectual decisions. They believe vision thus plays a decisive role in how we move, coordinate, think, and solve problems. . . .
>
> —Ann and Townsend Hoopes,
> *Eye Power*, p. 43.
>
> Furthermore, for the physicist, the whole question of the structure of matter is studded with paradoxes. Light, the very substance that allows people to perceive external objects, is believed to behave both as a wave and as a particle—as both energy and matter. Also, the physicist now believes that time is relative to the speed at which an observer is moving. He no longer recognizes one fixed external reality; he believes that a perceived reality is inseparable from the mind of the observer.
>
> —Mike Samuels, M.D., and Nancy Samuels,
> *Seeing with the Mind's Eye*, p. 8.
>
> Scientists have continued to believe that the autonomic nervous system is beyond conscious control. Recent studies, however, have shown that control over the autonomic nervous system can be learned.
>
> —Mike Samuels, M.D., and Nancy Samuels,
> *Seeing with the Mind's Eye*, p. 222.

In *Journey to Ixtlan* by Carlos Castaneda, there is an interesting passage that illustrates the influence of the mind on one's self-image. Basically what don Juan attempted to show Carlos was that his own inner messages, which in Carlos's case were mainly self-critical and negative, were what kept him from succeeding at the tasks the old man set for him; and that by changing these messages—"lying" to himself, as don Juan said, i.e., telling himself how good and worthwhile he was—Carlos could change the outcome.

Much the same is true in doing the Bates work: your inner expectations may strongly affect your progress. If you deeply believe that you can improve your vision, that you deserve to have perfect eyesight, then part of the battle is already won; you will probably make good progress. But if, while believing these things, you also constantly rely on your glasses, constantly underscore your disability with inner messages such as: *I can't see*; *my eyes are bad*; *my vision is terrible;* or if you feel strong embarrassment when you cannot read a menu without your glasses or do not recognize a friend sitting across the room at a gathering, then, to some degree, you undermine your progress.

"I already know that you think you are rotten," he said. "That's your *doing*. Now in order to affect that *doing* I am going to recommend that you learn another *doing*. From now on, and for a period of eight days, I want you to lie to yourself. Instead of telling yourself the truth, that you are ugly and rotten and inadequate, you will tell yourself that you are the complete opposite, knowing that you are lying and that you are absolutely beyond hope."

"But what would be the point of lying like that, don Juan?"

"It may hook you to another *doing* and then

> you may realize that both *doings* are lies, unreal, and that to hinge yourself to either one is a waste of time, because the only thing that is real is the being in you that is going to die. To arrive at that being is the *not-doing* of the self."
>
> —Carlos Castaneda,
> *Journey to Ixtlan*, Pocket Books, 1975, p. 20.

A kind of self-hypnosis. A constant stream of thoughts of illness, unworthiness, poor eyesight, catastrophes; of memories of bad events, of what you did wrong; in short, an emphasis upon the negative, is like feeding information into a computer, only in this case, the computer is you. With such a program, what can you expect to result?

Each of us is different, and some of us may have a basically positive attitude with only a few negative areas, one of which may be vision. So simply watch your thoughts as if they were characters in a film. Let them parade by, expressing themselves so that you get to know them. Let them just occur, and take note of what you emphasize.

Once you are aware of how you think, you might begin to probe for the reasons behind the negative thoughts. Then try an experiment. Take just one of your negative attitudes—a small one—and work toward replacing it. By "work" I suggest simply relaxing for another five minutes each day, and during that time "lie" to yourself, tell yourself that the exact opposite—and what you desire—is true.

For example, let's say you constantly tell yourself how tired you are. And, in fact, you *are* tired, as you will no doubt protest. For the five-minute period, tell yourself—and, for this few minutes, put your whole being into *believing* your "lie"—*I have a lot of energy and stamina.* Then go about your business as usual without paying any more attention to the matter. You might also do something symbolic of the new idea—go for a brisk walk, get up five minutes earlier, or go to bed five minutes later than usual—something that puts muscle behind the new thought. Be careful how you phrase your thought—it should always be in positive terms. To say, *I am not tired*, only reinforces the idea of fatigue.

Next, repeat the above exercise for your vision. Tell yourself, my vision is perfect, clear, and easy, or any variation that pleases you, so long as it is positive. You visualize yourself without glasses, imagining yourself comfortable doing and seeing what you now cannot do or see without them. As an activity to reinforce the exercise, go without your glasses sometimes, as long as you are comfortable.

The above exercise is a mind-to-body exercise, aimed at changing the inner self-image that maintains your poor vision. Your self-image creates the person you are (*I am what I think I am*), keeps you healthy or ill, rich or poor, happy or miserable. External events in themselves are not really so different for people as they may seem. But what *is* different is an individual's interpretation and response to those events. While one person will take an event as a challenge, another will view it as a defeat. Once you understand that you really do control that response and that interpretation, then you will recognize that you are in control of those events, and not the other way around. Until you are in control of your own health and vision, until you accept responsibility for them, then you will feel yourself a victim of outside forces—bad eyes, heredity, etc.—and you will not be able to change them significantly.

Once you understand your own power, then altering your vision will become a very real and positive challenge. So begin by gently and gradually replacing your negative beliefs and thoughts about your vision. Send your body the proper message: *My vision is clear and easy.* Once again, be careful after the five-minute period that you do not simply bury your negative thoughts and feelings. Respect them; they are there and part of you. To become positive beyond what you can realistically accomplish can backfire with a vengeance! And the denial of negative thoughts can be, oddly, a reinforcement of them; when you are afraid to allow them, to express them, it is because you believe them to be more powerful than their opposites. So do the exercise for only five minutes once a day. Otherwise, just observe your thoughts.

To change takes time; don't expect miracles. You have been programming your poor vision for some time; you once had reasons for doing so, though those reasons may not be immediately available to you. It is not necessary to go looking for those reasons. By looking for what went *wrong,* you would continue to pursue the negative. You live in the present, and it is in the here and now that change occurs.

Journal Entry

January 8, 1977

It's as though I edit what comes in. A selection is made, so my eyes jump from one thing to another, even within an individual object. Only what I feel is *important* is allowed, as if I'm trying to grasp what's out there in pieces so I can *control* what's there. That's in my mind. Control is put on the eyes to just take in pieces with large gaps left out. Doing swings, as I let it all come in, I feel my whole body relax, feel more energy available.

This next exercise, also to be done for only five minutes, uses a body-to-mind approach. Simply stand comfortably, with your eyes closed, and let yourself become aware of your body posture. Stand near a wall or piece of furniture so you can catch your balance if need be. Relax. In your imagination feel your muscles all over, moving your consciousness over your body like a radar screen. Make no judgments; just notice and feel how you stand. You may wish to make adjustments; do so being sure they are adjustments that come from a real desire within, and not from the usual childhood admonitions, the "shoulds" of posture such as, "straighten up," "pull in your tummy," etc. Your body will teach you its own needs. It will move, with your cooperation, toward its own balance. Respect your body; let it tell you what it needs, then follow through. The mind and body, working together, supporting each other, make a powerful combination. Use them in a unity, not one against the other, then see the results!

CHAPTER 6
Let's see

Chapter 7 will outline a Bates program, one you can follow if you are nearsighted, farsighted, astigmatic, or have developed middle-age sight. But before going into the exercises themselves, let us glance at the rationale behind them and some of the basic theories that Dr. Bates discovered.

Relaxation

Relaxation is fundamental to all of the Bates exercises. Tension and an anxiety or strain to see are the culprits causing poor vision; consequently their opposites—relaxation and ease—are the desired ends. Relaxation is not difficult to achieve, but it is a state of being you must *want*. You may have become so used to an inner state of tension that you may not even be aware that you are tense. You may also simply prefer that state, strange as that might sound, because it is familiar; change sometimes causes anxiety in people even when the change is for the better. So remember: you always *can* relax, but sometimes you may not *want* to. When you accept that idea, you accept responsibility for your state of being.

> The body exhibits a group of general changes every time relaxation takes place. Dr. Benson postulates that learning to relax voluntarily may have a role in treating diseases, such as hypertension, that are caused by prolonged excitation of the sympathetic nervous system.
>
> —Mike Samuels, M.D., and Nancy Samuels, *Seeing with the Mind's Eye*, p. 222.

Relaxation is a total condition. It is impossible to relax only your eyes, for example, and the Bates exercises aim at total relaxation. Always be aware of your whole body; if tension exists in one part, it will spill over into others. As you do the exercises, inventory your body, making sure that you maintain softness and smoothness. When you notice an area of tightness, pause and relax that part again. This is not really as difficult as it might sound, but initially, you will need to pay careful attention in order to break long-standing habits. Notice particularly your neck, shoulders, and face.

There are two types of relaxation. One is a complete letting-go, as, for example, when you soak in a hot tub. The other is what Huxley calls "dynamic relaxation." This is the kind of physical and mental fluidity with which we all would ideally function. It is perhaps best illustrated by athletes or dancers. In order to run or ski or leap effectively and gracefully, both body and mind must be receptive and flexible, not taut and rigid. Good dancers and athletes move with an ease that comes from a trained, but relaxed, body and mind.

Journal Entry

April 28, 1977

All this time—a year and a half—while I've sensed that fear was behind my visual problem, I probed psychologically, looking for frightening or traumatic experiences that created the fear and consequent withdrawal of vision. There were a number of things I could pin it on, but it all didn't quite *fit*. Last night I understood deeply. It was *seeing itself* I was afraid of!!! Bates has said it, I'd read it all, but I hadn't really understood. . . . Normal attention occurs in a relaxed state. The person can be attentive to the center of what's going on, yet allow the periphery, the outside events and happenings to enter without losing the center, letting the mind wander freely. But intense concentration cuts off external stimuli, pulls inward, results in tension. Forced, and by forced I mean self-inflicted force, concentration results in greater tension and the tendency to stare. The stare creates the blur. True *vision*, letting peripheral information also come in, became a thing of danger, of distraction, a temptation to me to let my attention wander, thus a thing to be avoided and feared. Seeing became my enemy. I had to *not* see, so I could direct my attention to Ms. Smith and her lessons. I admired her, liked her and was pleased she liked me, that I was doing well.

When vision is perfect, the mind and eyes are *receptors*, and they are relaxed. The eyes move easily and rapidly over the surface and edges of the object viewed; the mind receives the impressions and sees. Relaxation exercises affect the mind by allowing the anxiety of the viewer to dissipate, permitting him or her to take in the external world without strain. When the mind lets go of the strain, the eyes do what comes naturally to them: the muscles relax, the eye globe resumes its normal shape, and vision occurs. These muscles are both voluntary and involuntary. We use the voluntary part of the muscles to move the eyeballs up, down, sideways. But where these muscles attach to the eyeball, they are involuntary, controlled by the autonomic nervous system, *not* by our conscious minds. Relaxed, these muscles function naturally and easily; tense, they lock into place, holding the eyeball rigid so that it can no longer accommodate for all distances. As you relax with the Bates exercises, these muscles will let go, sometimes suddenly, resulting in a moment of perfectly clear or improved vision called a flash. More often, the muscles will let go gradually, so that you notice improvements over a period of months.

Nearly all the Bates exercises are relaxing. But since every person is unique, the exercises can have different effects on different people. Only you can judge which exercises are the most relaxing, and thereby most beneficial, to you. Let what makes you feel *good* guide you to the most helpful exercises. Be on guard against strain, against your habit of wanting to achieve. Vision simply comes, like a gift. If you strain for it, try too hard, become tense and anxious about it, you will defeat yourself. So relax. Do the exercises without testing yourself, without the sense that vision is your *goal*. Relaxation is your goal. The vision will take care of itself.

Movement

The second directive behind all the Bates exercises is to break the habit of staring by getting movement back into the mind and eyes. Movement and relaxation go together: the more relaxed you are, the smoother, the easier the movement. But initially, whether you are relaxed or not, it is essential to restore movement to the eyes. All of the exercises emphasize this principle, either actually or through the imagination; because movement results in "shifting," which means that your eyes move rapidly all over an object, taking in its many details. Shifting is not something you can accomplish with effort. It comes of its own, with relaxation, and with it, comes vision.

All of life consists of movement. When movement stops, life stops. You need think only of a river that stagnates when it is stopped up; or of a tree that stands dead and stiff in the midst of its flowing, moving brothers. A stare is nonmovement. It can be likened to holding a muscle taut. Can you imagine holding your arm stiff in one position for even 15 minutes? It would *hurt*. Yet you hold your eyes that way when you stare. When your eyes fix in a stare, they stop seeing, and the world blurs.

Staring, however, is a habit, and habits, as we know, are notoriously hard to break. Your nose will help you break the habit. Dr. Bates said, "When you want to see something, point your nose at it." You use your nose, quite literally, because it will be some time before you can trust your eyes to move for you, so when the instruction is given to "follow" your nose, do so quite seriously. Your nose will help bring movement back to you.

Psychologists have found that if a person's gaze becomes absolutely fixed while looking at an object, the image of the object will extinguish within seconds. Most people are unfamiliar with this phenomenon because in the course of normal seeing they unconsciously move their eyes continuously. Studies have shown that people move

> their eyes in small, jerky scanning movements even when they are looking at an object that is not moving. If a person fixes his gaze on a mental image, it likewise tends to disappear. Whereas if a person scans a mental image as if it were a perception, he will find the image tends to be clearer and more stable. . . .
>
> A person can only see the foreground or the distance clearly—never both at once. . . . If a person closes his eyes and tries to visualize a ball as it would appear two feet in front of him, but "mentally" focuses as if the ball were across the room, his mental image will be fuzzy and unclear.
>
> —Mike Samuels, M.D., and Nancy Samuels, *Seeing with the Mind's Eye*, p. 59.
>
> Life reveals itself most plainly when you do not clutch at it, neither with your feelings, or with your questing intellect. Touch and go. This is the whole art. That's why our eyes see best when they brush across things and do not stare in a fixed gaze. Everything kept goes stale. And the reason is, that whatever is momentous, living and moving, is momentary. Minute by minute, our experience moves along without return, and we are in accord with it to the degree that we move with it as the mind follows music or as a leaf goes with the stream.
>
> —Alan Watts, *Haiku*, a recording by Musical Engineering Associates, 1959.

Centralization

The healthy, seeing eye/mind sees clearly only one small point of any object viewed. The size of this point is about the same as the head of a pin! Because the eyes and mind move with such rapidity, the viewer has the illusion that he sees everything at once. People with poor vision have lost this ability to centralize—i.e. to see one point clearly and all other points less well. A couple of exercises in centralization are included mainly to bring about an awareness of it. Centralization is one of the gifts of clear vision; it occurs with relaxation. If you pay too much attention to it, centralization will elude you because you will be straining for it. You need only know about it, then relax and let it happen on its own.

Fusion

Because we have two eyes, we also have two pictures of what we observe. The brain takes these two images and puts them together to make one. This process is called fusion because the two images are fused.

Sometimes, however, the muscles around one or even both eyes fail to work together so that the two eyes are pointed at different objects, as, for example, in crossed eyes. The eye or eyes may go in or out, or up or down; in any case the condition is known as squint. In squint, there are two separate images, which the mind cannot fuse since two completely different parts of an object are being seen simultaneously. The result is double vision, which the mind cannot tolerate. What happens? Literally, the mind turns off one of the eyes—like unscrewing a light bulb. The person sees then with only one eye, with the resultant loss of depth perception. In many cases of squint, simple exercises can be used to correct the condition. In any case, two fusion exercises are included for those without squint because fusion can always be improved. High myopes (people with a high degree of nearsightedness) tend toward a loss of fusion. The exercises can prevent this loss before it takes hold.

> If you are myopic . . . most optometrists will prescribe minus lenses. . . . This will improve your sharpness and clarity, but it will also narrow your scope of vision. . . . Depending on their strength, minus lenses provide the kind of vision you use when you aim a rifle; it is clear and sharp, but narrowly concentrated, and it produces stress for just those reasons. By reducing your field of vision, minus lenses also reduce your capacity to absorb experience visually. By overemphasizing central vision and attenuating peripheral vision, they can adversely affect bodily balance and general coordination, for it is peripheral vision that provides the frame or context for the objects you see; without it, you experience difficulty in precisely locating yourself in space. . . . It is the strength and efficiency of your peripheral vision that permits you to judge the true size of, and thus the true spatial relationship between, the various objects in the central field.
>
> —Ann and Townsend Hoopes,
> *Eye Power*, Alfred A. Knopf, 1979, pp. 95, 98.

Reading

Reading is so much a part of our lives that whether you are nearsighted, farsighted, or astigmatic, you can benefit from the reading techniques and practices that Dr. Bates and his followers developed. Reading should be comfortable and pleasurable, but for many people it is neither, and can even be a source of acute pain. With relaxation, good light, and movement, the possibility of reading with comfort can be realized. For farsighted people and those with middle-age-sight, this is especially good news. Just remember: as with any vision improvement, *relaxation comes first*. If you only concentrate on the reading exercises, or rush through the others in order to do them, you will be defeating yourself. The early exercises in the Bates program are the most important ones because they are the most relaxing ones.

CHAPTER 7

The common disorders: For the nearsighted, farsighted, astigmatic, and those with middle-age sight

The exercises that follow are arranged into weekly lessons to be done over a period of three months. After the initial lesson, you will add only one or two new things each week. The *familiarity* of the exercises is important—the more familiar an exercise is, the more relaxed you will be with it. Progress in vision training is measured in degrees of relaxation, not in the numbers of exercises you do.

WARNING: People with special vision defects, such as glaucoma, cataracts, etc., should first read the sections in Chapter 8 that deal specifically with these disorders. In any case, *people with such disorders should first consult their ophthalmologist before embarking on any program.*

General Instructions

The Bates Method is a reconditioning process. Like jogging, it benefits you only if you do it consistently. If you jog only once a week, you might end up doing yourself more harm than good. You can never harm yourself practicing the Bates Method, but you will probably not make much progress if you do not apply yourself every day. Practice as much as possible. If you have a busy schedule, find or create one time slot a day for the exercises, then pay particular attention to the suggestions given for integrating the exercises into your daily life.

Always remove your glasses during the exercises, and go without them as much as you can. Put them on, however, when you feel strain or discomfort. Never go without glasses while driving, until you have passed the motor vehicle vision test without glasses. But you will find many times throughout the day when you can slip them off and still feel comfortable. Use such moments.

Contact lens wearers must change back to glasses. Contacts defeat the Bates work because they themselves cause tension in the eyes.

It is best if you can have a pair of weaker glasses—a correction of 20/40 rather than 20/20. Or you may want to use an older pair of glasses with a weaker correction than your present pair. These will allow your eyes flexibility, a chance to hold on to a small improvement that you might not notice. Putting on your 20/20 glasses forces your eyes to adjust back to the weaker condition in order to see through the lenses.

Never wear sunglasses or tinted lenses of any kind. With the sunning exercises, your eyes will soon accustom themselves to bright light. If you are extremely light-sensitive, you can use a hat with a visor in the early weeks.

Learn to relax with the blur when you aren't wearing your glasses. And recognize how much you *can* see even if it is blurred. Look around you. Look out the window. You may miss details in the distance or close up, but you can no doubt identify many of the objects beyond the point where you think you can no longer see.

You may experience "funny" sensations—watering eyes, twinges, tickles in and around your eyes. None of these should be unpleasant. If you experience headaches, pain, or any discomfort, then you are probably not following directions, or are straining for results. Dr. Bates said, "Any *effort* you make to see will result in failure." And Huxley said, "Seeing is effortless." Ignore your vision for a while. Just be aware of your varying levels of tension and relaxation.

Lesson 1, First Week

1. Massage and breathe
2. Sun
3. Palm
4. Easy open, easy close
5. Blinking

1. Massage and breathe

Sit in a chair with your feet flat on the floor, hands resting softly in your lap. Sit erectly with your back straight but not rigid. Close your eyes. Take a deep breath through your nose and let it out through your mouth with a sigh. Do this two or three times. Now, with your eyes still closed, slowly begin to massage your cheeks with your fingers, using a circular motion.

Be aware of how good it feels. Now massage your temples, using the same circular movement. Every once in a while, take a deep breath and let it out with a sigh. Massage your forehead next, then your whole scalp. Take your time with this exercise. There is no hurry. Now cap your hands over your head, as illustrated below, and, using your thumbs, press and massage the two hollows at the base of your skull.

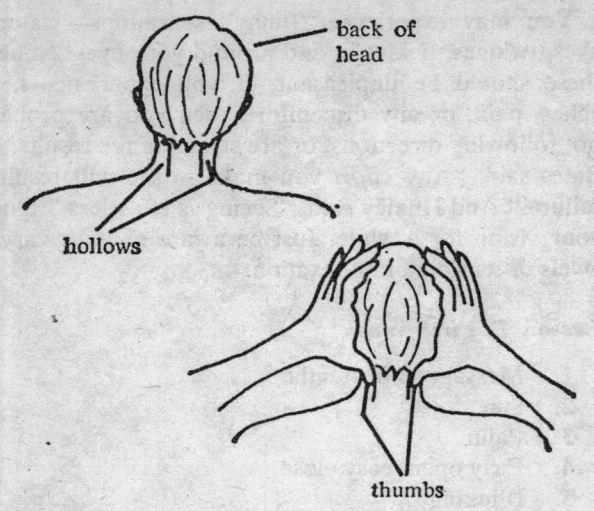

place hands like this ...

If these are tender, massage gently.

Be aware of your arms. If they need a rest or shaking out, then rest them or shake them. Remember: if you have tension in one part of your body, you will have tension in other parts as well. Also be aware of your breathing. Relaxed, you breathe deeply and easily; tense, you breathe shallowly, or even hold your breath. Notice how you breathe throughout the day—it is an indicator of relaxation and tension.

Now, using your index and middle fingers, lift and drop the muscle that runs just above the eyebrow. Alternately lift one side as you drop the other (right eye, left eye), so that you get a rocking movement.

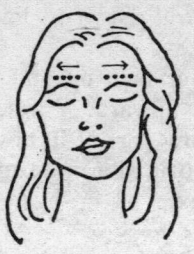
dots indicate the muscle

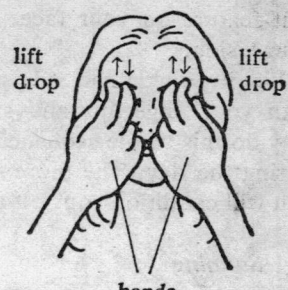
hands

Start in the middle of your forehead and work out in a straight line to the top of your ear. Return to the middle and move outward again. Repeat ten to twenty times. Go slowly. Always take your time.

Next, gently press and release all around the bony ridge that encircles your eyes. Use your thumbs along the upper ridge, your index finger along the lower ridge.

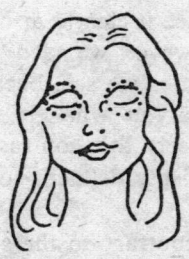
dots represent the bony ridge

You may find some sore spots. Be gentle with these, and the soreness will gradually work itself out.

Now massage your nose—thoroughly. This may make it necessary for you to blow your nose. Over the next few weeks, your nose will become the most important feature on your face. You will use it to improve your vision.

Finally, tickle the sides of your face up and down with your fingertips and stretch upward. Yawn. You may do this whole sequence, or any part of it, any time during the day. The more you do it, the more quickly you will condition yourself to relax.

2. *Sunning*

In any number of ancient cultures, the day began with a sun greeting, where breath (often in a chant) and light conjoined in a ritual act that asserted that breath and light *were* life. In many religions and cultures, the sun was God, or the Source. In terms of vision, light is certainly the source. Without it, we see only shadings of gray and black. In fact, certain of the cells composing the retina—the rods—specifically facilitate this kind of seeing, for night vision and vision in dim light. Because the rods are most concentrated off from the center of the retina, we need to look off slightly to one side of an object in order to see it clearly at night or in dim light.

To see color, however, we need light, and the brighter the light, the better we see, because then there is a sharp contrast between what is lit and what is in shadow. It is precisely this contrast that makes seeing easy, with edges crisply defined, colors brightly delineating forms.

In our culture, contrary to the sun-worshipping cultures, light is shunned, other than for sun-bathing. We stay indoors, drive vehicles with tinted glass, wear dark glasses, even build windowless structures where no sun penetrates; all the indoor light is provided artificially, most commonly by fluorescent fixtures that cast only the dimmest of shadows. People become light-sensitive, unable to be comfortable outside in natural sunlight.

Yet the eyes are organs of light; deprived of it, they cease to see at all—in short, they go blind. Wearing sunglasses to "protect" the eyes from natural light is like wearing earmuffs to "protect" the ears from the songs of birds. What a strange world we have evolved!

And increasing evidence is showing that the light is necessary not only to our eyes and vision, but to our overall health as well. John Ott's informative and highly readable book, *Health and Light,* graphically describes some of the effects of light deprivation in both human beings and animals. Light, as he illustrates, means the full spectrum of natural sunlight taken in through the naked eye, not through plastic or glass lenses that cut out some of the spectrum.

Through the sunning exercise that follows, you will quickly reaccustom yourself to natural sunlight. The sun itself is, of course, the best source of light in which to do this exercise, but the sun may not always be available, or your eyes may be such that you need to start with a lesser source of light and warmth. You may use the light described below, or even a smaller wattage bulb until you feel comfortable with the stronger light and/or the sun.

The problem of what to do [about his arthritis] continued to become more acute; then, one day I broke my glasses. While waiting for a new pair to be made, I wore my spares. The nose piece was a little tight and it bothered me, so I took them off most of the time. The weather had been nice for several days, and there was some light work outside that I did as best I could with my cane in one hand. Suddenly I didn't seem to need the cane. My elbow was fine, and my hip was not bothering me much, even though I hadn't taken any extra amount of aspirin. It was hard to figure out why my arthritis should suddenly be so much better.

My hip hadn't felt this well for three or four years. . . .

My particular reason for not wearing dark glasses was that in addition to the glass itself filtering out virtually all the ultraviolet and certain other shorter wavelengths of sunlight energy, the characteristics of the light are further changed depending on the color of the glass. . . .

Theories may be interesting to think about and discuss with other people, but this was affecting my own arthritis, a much more personal and realistic matter. Maybe I was one of the lucky people you hear about who get better for no reason at all, but I felt strongly that there was a reason. I had taken my glasses off and let the full unfiltered natural sunlight energy into my eyes and had also made a point of being outdoors six hours or more each day whether it was sunny or cloudy. To me the results were convincing enough; the light received through the eyes must stimulate the pituitary or some other gland such as the pineal gland about which not too much is known. . . .

After six months of not wearing glasses, except for what little driving of the car was absolutely essential . . . I began to notice that wearing my glasses . . . seemed to strain my eyes more and more. Accordingly, an appointment with my oculist . . . seemed advisable. This time it was necessary to go back for a second examination which my doctor explained was customary in order to double check any such drastic change as was the case with the condition of my eyes. The principal difference in my new prescription was that the rather strong prisms previously needed to correct a muscular weakness were no longer needed. With this encouragement, I decided also to have my hip X-rayed. . . .

It was most gratifying to have my doctor advise that the X-ray pictures showed a definite strengthening and improvement in the area of my hip joint. . . . A physical examination revealed the complete disappearance of a 30 percent restriction of the movement or rotation of the hip

> joint which my doctor commented on as being wonderful but quite surprising and most unusual.
>
> —John N. Ott,
>   *Health and Light,* Pocket Books, 1977, pp. 58–69.

The Sunning Lamp Use a 150-watt indoor reflector spotlight in a ceramic socket. (The plastic and metal sockets get too hot.) If you have a goose-neck lamp, this will work very well. Otherwise you can buy a clamp attachment, which usually includes the ceramic socket, in the electrical department of a hardware store. This can then be clamped onto a chair.

WARNING: *Never* sun with your eyes open. Always sun for short periods, no more than ten minutes at a time, and again, *never* use a "sun lamp." Use the lamp described above, or the sun. Position the light at whatever distance is comfortable for you. You have to be your own judge here. If you feel strain, or want to squint, then the light's too close. It should never feel too hot or too bright. If it does, move it back. Sunning is a pleasant exercise, not one you should feel you are enduring. If you are especially light-sensitive, begin with a lower-watt bulb, working gradually to the spotlight. Outdoors, you might need to begin by sitting in the shade at first, then in the sun with your eyes downward until you get used to the brightness. Don't worry about how "fast" you accustom yourself. Your eyes will gradually regain the joy of the light. Take your time. Be aware of how you feel.

Your Nose Because your eyes are accustomed to staring, to a certain rigidity, you will use your nose to help you regain mobility. You cannot trust your eyes to move, but you can trust your nose, because moving it includes moving your whole head. Thus you will know whether or not you are moving. All you have to do then is to allow your seeing to follow where your nose is pointing. Remember: "When you want to see something, point your nose at it."

To help you further, use your imagination. Imagine that you have a magical fiber attached to the end of your nose that can reach out to any distance, can touch and feel things, can write or paint; in fact, imagine that it can do anything you want it to do. Always be aware of this fiber and allow your attention to follow it.

The Exercise Now, with your light on, (or facing the sun), *your eyes closed*, take a deep breath. Welcome the light inside your head. Let it fill up the inside of your head with its warmth and energy. Remember that your eyes thrive on light and need it just as your body needs food.

Use the fiber on the end of your nose and, moving your head in a circle to move the fiber, slowly begin drawing a circle around the sun or light. Let your attention follow the fiber. Draw a few circles, then reverse direction and draw a few the other way. Now imagine that the light has become a big daisy five feet in front of you. Feel the petals moving past as you draw a circle around the flower. Be aware of the whiteness of the petals, the yellow center. Reverse directions.

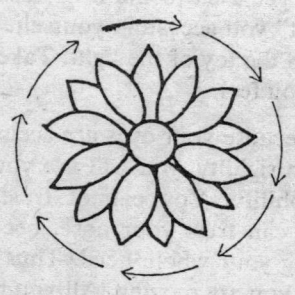

Take your time, enjoy the warmth of the sun. Yawn. Breathe. This first week, only sun for a few minutes several times a day. After you circle the daisy, point your nose fiber to the far left, and write your first name in big letters, in any color you choose, across the light. Turn off your light or move out of the sun into shade.

3. Palming

Palming is the opposite of sunning—i.e., all light is cut off from the eyes and mind, giving the visual system a complete rest. The hands are placed over the closed eyes, bringing warmth and energy to them. Palming can be done anytime, anywhere, for as long as you want. You may lie down, pillows on your chest to support your arms, and simply listen to music or the daily sounds around you. Or, you may sit, your elbows resting on a pillow on a table, or with pillows in your lap, and do a palming exercise, two of which are included in this chapter. But the most relaxing thing you can do while palming is to *remember*. Dr. Bates discovered that the recall of pleasant memories was one of the most relaxing things a person could do, and urged his patients to use their own memories during palming. The main thing here is that the memories be pleasant; if you sit and worry you will end up a wreck!

The Exercise Pile some pillows on your lap so you can rest your elbows on them, or sit at a table with a pillow under your elbows. Or, lie down as described above. Now place the palms of your hands over your eyes. The base of your hands should rest more or less on your cheekbones; your palms will form a hollow over your closed eyes. One hand will rest on top of the other on your forehead. There should be no pressure on your eyes; you can open them, although you will keep them closed during the exercise. Keep your hands soft and relaxed, and avoid pinching your nose. Although ideally you should see total darkness, a little light slipping in here and there is preferable to your tensing your hands and arms or squeezing your nose so that you cannot breathe. With adjustments and a little practice, your palming technique will improve.

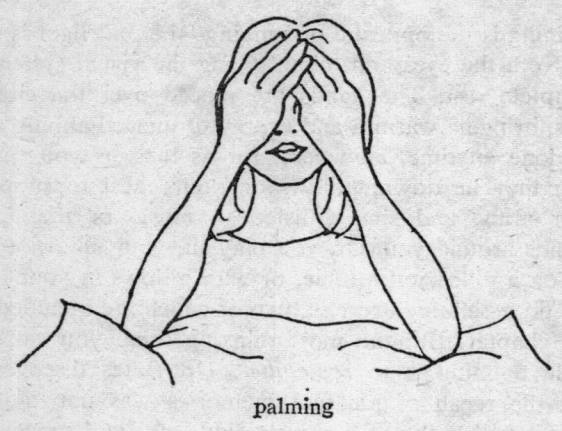

palming

Now simply rest and use your memory to return to a place and time when you were very comfortable and happy. Recall *sounds, odors*, and *physical sensations*, such as the feel of the sun or wind, or your own body movements. Recall *textures, colors, objects,* and *shapes*. You might choose to return to a childhood spot or to a recent vacation place. Be alone; you want to avoid the stimulation of another's imagined presence. Your own personal, pleasant memories will induce the greatest relaxation. Palm for at least ten minutes. The longer, however, the better, *if* you remain relaxed.

4. Easy Open, Easy Close

The eyes love light, and they love the interplay of light and shadow. You will notice the greatest improvement in your vision outdoors on a bright, sunny day. But the eyes like a *gradual* transition from darkness into light, so always end the palming exercise with this one.

Keep your eyes closed, and lower your hands from palming. Keep your gaze directed downward toward your lap, and swing your head from side to side, *letting* your eyes come open briefly, *letting* them close again. Easy open, easy close. Do this until you feel quite comfortable with the brightness of the light.

5. Blinking

Blinking creates a movement on the retina by shutting off the image for a split second so that a fresh image appears when the blink is over. Such a movement is restful to both eyes and mind. Blinking breaks the stare, if only briefly, and should be the easiest thing in the world to do; yet it may be quite difficult for some people. Blinking is *not* closing one's eyes. It is a rapid, gentle movement.

Put your hands together as if in prayer. Let your hands be very soft, the tips of your fingers just barely touching.

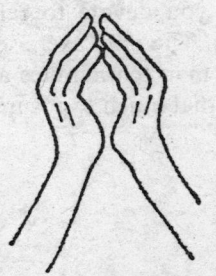

Hands like a butterfly

You have seen a butterfly on a flower, its wings upright, similar to the way you now hold your hands. Its wings open, then close, touching ever so slightly. Imagine that your hands are the wings of a butterfly. Touch your fingertips together gently and briefly. Barely touch them, moving your fingertips back immediately upon sensing the delicate touch. Do this with your eyes closed, so that you feel it at first. Establish a rhythm. Touch—inhale slowly and deeply, then exhale—touch—breathe again to help time yourself—touch. Now open your eyes, and each time you touch your fingers together, blink—continue your breathing—blink—blink. Let your breathing be the space between your blink/touch. And remember, blinking is not closing the eyes. It is a rapid, and eventually, unconscious, movement. For now, you will have to constantly be on the alert about blinking. Remind yourself, asking yourself, *Am I blinking?* This first week, be especially aware that you want to establish this as a habit.

Summary

This week, 1) massage once or twice a day for at least ten minutes; 2) sun a couple of minutes twice a day; 3) palm once for a minimum of at least twenty minutes; 4) blink all the time.

The more time you devote to relaxing, the sooner you will get results. The only exercise you must limit is sunning—no more than ten minutes at a time, provided your skin can take that much exposure.

Journal Entries

May 4 1977

This morning, for the first time, I felt a doubt rise. Am I fooling myself thinking this will really work? What followed shortly after, as I crossed the bridge, was a clearing that kept coming and going all morning, in waves. It's no longer flashes, but waves of clearing—the clarity lasting longer and leaving more slowly—also the *feeling* again, of something familiar as from a long time ago; a feeling of permitting everything to enter, a softness in my body, all over.

May 6, 1977

How hard it is to break the stare, the old way of seeing. I know it takes a lot of effort to block vision, yet the lure of what's known and familiar keeps perpetuating the blur. I sense what I have to do, but sometimes feel frustrated by it, almost defeated.

May 16, 1977

Driving down Snelling today, my vision cleared a *lot*, and held for maybe five-ten minutes. Eyes felt different, a pressure on either side. Don't know if that was straining or not, but it was also a feeling of *looking* with curiosity.

Lesson 2, Second Week

1. Sun
2. Palm
3. Massage and breathe
4. The long swing
5. The ball toss

1. Sun

Sun as before—eyes closed, facing the sun or light. Take a deep breath and welcome the light. Let it fill the inside of your head. Imagine that you are tiny and that you sit inside your head, way at the back of your skull. Your eyes are two large windows with the shades drawn over them. The light passes through these windows back to where you sit.

Circle the light with your nose, as before. Always move your head, and let your attention casually follow where your nose fiber touches. Let the light become a daisy now, and circle it in both directions.

Now imagine that there is a picket fence out in front of you.

Nearsighted People Imagine that the picket fence is two feet in front of you. The fence is about three feet high, made of wood and freshly painted white. The sun is behind you and shines directly on the fence. Point your nose to the left side of the fence. Drag your fiber through the pickets from left to right. *Feel* the pickets ticking by on the end of your nose fiber. *Hear* the sound your fiber makes—similar to the sound a stick would make if dragged across the surface of the fence. *Notice* how the pickets seem to be moving. As you drag your fiber from the left side across to the right, the pickets seem to move to the left. As you swing back from right to left, the pickets appear to move to the right. The movement of the pickets is always opposite to the movement of your head. (If you have trouble imagining this movement, think of how it looks on the movie screen when the camera suddenly moves across the scenery—you are aware then not of the camera moving, but of the scenery rapidly moving past.) Swing your nose from side to side several times.

Now let the fence drift off. Imagine it is across the

street from you or across the yard, about 25 to 30 feet away. Continue to swing your nose fiber along the pickets, noticing, feeling, and hearing the oppositional movement.

Let the fence drift off further into the distance. It is tiny because it is so far away—about one city block away, on top of a grassy green hill. Your peripheral vision tells you that green fields surround you. The fence is silhouetted against the bright blue sky. Continue swinging your head from side to side.

Farsighted People Read through the above exercise, then do it exactly the same way, but begin with the picket fence off in the distance and gradually move it in closer until it is two feet in front of you.

End your sunning exercise by writing your first name in big letters across the light. Choose a color for the letters, and follow the point of your nose as it forms each letter.

2. Palm

Palm as before for at least ten minutes. Finish palming with the easy open, easy close exercise.

3. Breathe and Massage

Now do the facial massage exactly as in Lesson 1. Take your time and breathe, sigh, yawn.

4. The Long Swing

"Swings" are wonderful for producing movement and developing an awareness of movement. They are also the most natural movements in the world, hence the most relaxing. Basically, a swing is a rocking motion, and since we all began by being rocked in our parents' arms, what could be more conducive to relaxation?

There are many kinds of swings; in fact, any movement you make constitutes a "swing," so long as you allow your attention to follow your nose.

If the weather permits, do the long swing outdoors; otherwise, do it in the largest room in your home so that you have the most space. Do it every day for a minimum count of 100, or for five to ten minutes. The longer you do it, the greater the benefit. And remember to *blink* and *breathe*.

Stand with your feet a little less than shoulder width apart. Throughout this exercise, keep your nose in a direct vertical line above your navel so that your spine remains straight, but *not* rigid. All movement occurs in the feet and legs. Let your arms hang freely.

the long swing

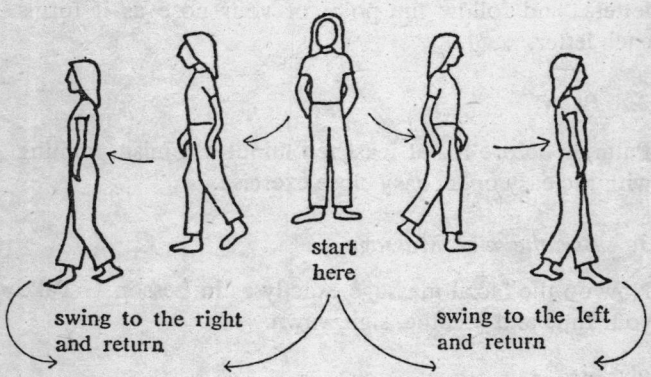

swing to the right and return

start here

swing to the left and return

Pivot on the ball of your left foot, turning to the right and allowing the heel of your left foot to come forward. Keep your nose above your navel. When you have turned a quarter of a circle to the left, swing back to the center, then pivot on your right foot and swing to the right as in the illustration. *Let everything move.* Swing rhythmically, smoothly, from side to side, forming a half-circle as you turn from right to left, left to right. Blink. Sometimes point your nose down at the floor or ground right in front of your feet, sometimes up at the sky or along the ceiling, or along any plane between the two. Let your eyes follow wherever your nose points.

Swing relatively quickly so that you are not tempted to "see." Everything will move by rapidly, too fast for you to stare.

Sometimes close your eyes as you swing, and just feel the rocking movement. Pay no attention to your eyes, or to seeing. Just get into the rhythm of the movement as you would, say, to a waltz. Breathe easily.

5. Ball Toss

You may use any kind of ball for this exercise, but the brightly colored soft rubber balls that children use are the best because of the size and color. Toss whatever ball you have from your right hand to your left, and back again, the way a juggler would. Just move your head with it, keeping your nose on the ball as you toss it back and forth. When the ball lands in your hand, blink. Be aware of your breathing.

For variety, you can play ball with another person, throwing it back and forth between you. Simply follow the rule: *Keep your nose on the ball.* And blink and breathe. And sometimes close your eyes and follow the ball in your imagination; in other words, play the game of toss in your mind.

The ball toss is relaxing as long as it is done in a spirit of fun. Its purpose is to get movement back into the mind and eyes, to break the habit of staring, and to achieve "shifting." You may do this exercise as often and for as long as you wish, provided you remain relaxed.

Remember that you can always see better with your eyes closed than with them open. When you can imagine something perfectly with your eyes closed, your eye muscles will be relaxed and functioning as if you were really seeing what you imagine. Once you can remember that perfect image with your eyes open, you will see the object clearly.

> **Journal Entry**
>
> *February 28, 1978*
>
> Perfect vision is coming—oh, how often have I said that! How often have I felt it was just a matter of days or weeks? And yet again, I feel it. It is just so easy, soft, and relaxed, and perfect vision keeps coming in all the time. Even tonight, driving back from school, after 6:00, in near darkness, without glasses, I could relax and see pretty well. The oddest thing is that I can't pin down exactly what it is, what's responsible. It seems to be all of it—relaxation, shifting, and centralization.

To integrate the exercises into your daily life, be aware always of blinking and breathing. Palm for a brief moment here and there throughout the day, particularly when changing from one activity to another. Sun briefly at a window, or as you leave a building, or as you wait at a bus stop. Close your eyes occasionally to rest them.

Lesson 3, Third Week

1. Sun
2. Palm
3. Massage

4. Corridor swing
5. Ball toss
6. Conversation swing

1. Sun

Sun as in Lesson 2, but add the following visualization exercise after you finish visualizing the picket fence.

Nearsighted People Imagine a stepladder about two feet in front of you. Point your fiber at the bottom step. Feel it. Drag your fiber up the steps to the top, noticing how, as you go up, the steps appear to move down. Now go down; the steps appear to move upward. Slide smoothly up and down the ladder. Hear the oppositional movement. Feel it. If visualizing is hard for you, be patient. It will come. Relax. Go back to what is easy to imagine. The main thing is to get movement, even in the imagination. You need to break the habit of staring, and you stare even with your eyes closed, which is why you must always visualize things in motion during sunning and palming.

Let the ladder drift off to an imagined house, across the street, or at some middle distance from you. Now it is an aluminum painter's ladder that leans against the side of the house. Drag your fiber up and down the rungs of the ladder. Notice the movement.

Let it drift off to the distance of a block or two away, and put it up against a taller building. Continue swinging up and down the ladder. Finish sunning by writing your name, as in lesson 2.

Farsighted People Reverse the above directions, starting with the ladder at the farthest point and moving it in toward you.

2. Palm

Palm as before.

3. Massage

Massage as before.

4. Corridor Swing

Do the long swing exactly as before, but hold your arms straight out in front of you as illustrated below. Direct your vision between your arms, which form the "corridor." Watch how everything flies by!

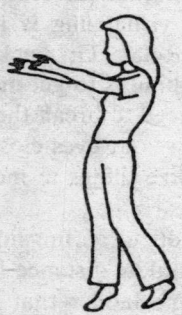

The Corridor Swing

The corridor swing helps you to keep your visual attention moving so that you do not "grab" things that pass by your line of vision. Alternate the corridor swing with the long swing so that your arms do not get tired or cramped.

5. Ball Toss

Do this as before.

6. Conversation Swing

People with poor vision, particularly nearsighted people, have an established habit of staring while talking with another person. The conversation swing helps to alleviate this problem. If you find it difficult at first, then practice on a photograph, on closeups of faces on TV, or in movies. Or even practice with your dog or cat. Then put the conversation swing into practice whenever you talk with someone.

As the speaker in a conversation, you can safely look away from your listener's face without appearing disinterested. Looking away is important because it is a *movement*, and movement is restful to the eyes and mind. Look up sometimes, away from your partner's face, as if searching for a word. Glance off to a distant object; close your eyes briefly. And, of course, blink. In other words, break the stare, and change your focus. *Use your nose*. Then, when you do focus on your partner's face, keep your nose moving so that you glide from one eye to the other, down the nose, around the mouth. This may be hard for you to do at first. Practice. At first the movements of your head as it follows your nose might be noticeable, but with practice, you will be able to keep your eyes shifting without anyone noticing what you are doing.

Journal Entry

August 14, 1978

To continue: My vision is holding somewhat, particularly out in this open country, but what's great is that it holds long enough to experience what normal vision is; thus, I am truly learning to see. In terms of this, I want to find the words to write a book to help others. I don't want the book to be an attack on the medical profession as others have

> suggested. To attack or place blame is also to give away your own authority. The essence of the Bates work is in recognizing your own power and how *you* screwed up, not someone else. The myope holds his vision in, focusing in front of large areas in an attempt to see all at once. Seeing clearly is allowing the center of vision to range freely over specific details. The whole is seen that way.

As the listener, you are more bound to maintain eye contact, so be careful to keep your nose moving around your partner's face. And whenever you get a chance, glance off. To fix eyes rigidly on one distance is like holding any muscle tightly in one position for a long period of time. What happens? The muscle aches. How to rest it? Movement. The eye muscles are no different. Restore the movement. The conversation swing is another exercise you can easily incorporate into your daily activities.

Lesson 4, Fourth Week

1. Sun
2. Palm
3. Massage and breathe
4. Long swing, corridor swing
5. Ball toss
6. Getting white
7. Driving swing

1 through 5

Do all of these exercises exactly as before.

6. Getting White

Dr. Bates discovered that there is no strain involved in looking at white, or at a solid-colored wall. To rest your eyes, and to prepare for chart work and reading, do the following exercise.

Close your eyes. Imagine that you are in the mountains standing at the base of a cliff. It is winter, and powdery white snow has recently fallen, covering the cliff in front of you. Breathe in the cold, fresh air. The sun is shining directly on the slope, making its new whiteness even whiter. Let your whole head fill up with this bright white.

Now sit facing a solid white wall, or hold up a piece of white paper in front of you at a comfortable distance. Just sit and regard the wall or paper. Blink. Breathe. Alternate opening your eyes on the whiteness, and closing your eyes and imagining the white slope.

7. Driving Swing

This is another exercise that can be integrated into your daily life. Use it every time you drive because driving is another situation in which we tend to stare. Of course, you must do this exercise with your glasses *on* if you need lenses to drive. *Never* drive without glasses until you pass the motor vehicle vision test without them.

Swing your nose from the gauges, to your rearview mirror, to the side mirror, and back to the road in front of you. Slowly swing your nose from side to side, from the line in the middle of the road to the right side and back. Swing from the horizon to closer in. Swing from a car close in front to one further off in the distance. Naturally, your swinging will depend somewhat on weather and traffic conditions. Be sure that you breathe and blink. The rule is always *Breathe, blink, swing*.

If you do not drive, then, as a passenger of either car or bus, take advantage of the movement around you. Just point your nose fiber out the window and let everything slide past. Relax with it; enjoy the movement.

Be aware of your tension and relaxation. If you wake up in a bad mood one day, or if you are having a rough time, then admit that you do not want to relax, and skip your exercises for the day. If you are relaxed, the exercises benefit you; if you are tense, they do you no good whatsoever.

Lesson 5, Fifth Week

1. Sun
2. Palm
3. Massage and breathe
4. Long swing, corridor swing
5. Ball toss
6. Yardstick swing
7. Getting white
8. Chart work

1 through 5

Do all of these exercises exactly as before.

6. Yardstick Swing

Obtain a wooden yardstick with the inches clearly marked off with black lines. Hardware stores often give these out when you buy paint, or sell them at a very reasonable cost. Sit down after the ball toss, and close your eyes briefly. Take a deep breath through your nose, and let it out with a sigh. Now hold your yardstick horizontally in front of you, about 10 to 15 inches away. Point your nose to the left of the yardstick, right on the edge of the stick itself. Drag your nose fiber along the edge of the stick to the right. Notice how the whole stick seems to move in the opposite direction in relation to the background. If it doesn't, then move the stick from side to side in the direction opposite to your movement as you swing your nose from left to right, right to left. Breathe, blink, and relax.

Now hold the stick vertically, and swing up and down, keeping your nose on the edge with the black lines. Again, simply notice the movement. As you swing up, the stick will appear to move down; as you swing down, it will appear to move up. When the stick is held horizontally, it will move the way your imagined picket fence moves; held vertically, it moves the way the imagined ladder moves.

Now hold the stick in the two diagonals, one after the other, as illustrated below. Do this exercise for as long as you remain relaxed. This exercise is especially good in helping to eliminate astigmatism. Sometimes close your eyes and imagine the yardstick moving in the opposite direction.

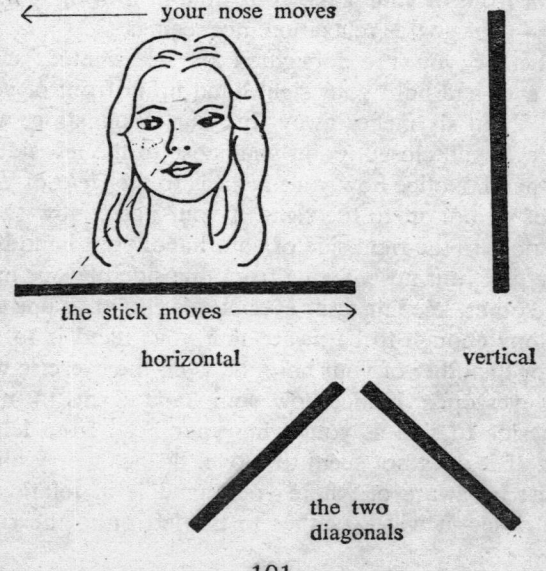

7. Getting White

Imagine the snowy white slope and work with your white paper or a wall.

8. Chart Work

You can obtain a Snellen eye chart from a medical supply store. It should be white, with the black letters printed upon it clearly.

Sit about 10 to 15 feet away from the chart. It does not matter whether or not you can see any of the letters, only that you be able to perceive the whiteness of the chart itself. If you feel uncomfortable at this distance, move to whatever distance feels good to you.

Farsighted People You may start the chart work with the chart at 10 to 15 feet, but gradually move it in close as you relax with the work until you have it about one foot in front of you. Take your time in moving it in so close—your goal is relaxation, not seeing.

Whether you are farsighted or nearsighted, close your eyes and hold your right hand up in front of your nose, about six inches away. In your imagination, with your eyes still closed, point your nose to the left side of your hand. Notice how your hand is to the *right* of your line of vision, or, to the right of your nose. Now swing your nose to the right side of your hand; your hand is to the *left* of your nose. Swing from one side of your hand to the other, keeping your eyes closed. Point to one side just long enough to be aware that your hand is to one side or the other of your nose. Now do the exercise with your eyes open. Notice how your hand seems to move from side to side as you swing your head from left to right. If it does not seem to move, do not worry about it; just be aware of where your hand is in relation to your nose—it will be either to the left or to the right.

Close your eyes again and, in your imagination, point your nose to the left side of the chart out in front of you. (You should mount your chart on a board and either place it so that the sunlight shines directly upon it or shine your sunning light on it.) Notice how the chart is to the right. Now swing to the other side. Where is the chart in relation to your nose? Swing from one side to the other, with your eyes still closed. When it is easy for you to imagine the swing with your eyes closed, then open them and continue the exercise. Just notice which side the chart is on in relation to your nose. Look as far to one side of the chart as you need in order to get the movement.

Journal Entries

February 5, 1979

I had a dream about seeing. I recall how the dream showed me how to "scan." Then last night—I was tired and resting—I practiced it. It's not so different from what Bates teaches, except I had some other awareness of the inner blocking that goes on. The awareness: the myope looks out on the world, looking for something—looks out the way a person in fear looks, blocking out everything except the object of fear at which he stares, fascinated. The blurring occurs, and what was once perhaps a response to a real stimulus— an object of fear, or a moment of fear—becomes a habit, useless, and an obstacle. As a child I had some fears—darkness especially—and I recall wanting to fall asleep before whatever was going to happen happened so that *I wouldn't have to see it*. When I begin to scan, I am *very* tight in my arms, shoulders, upper back, and neck; my breathing is also tight. The original resistance to seeing I had so long ago continues.

July 12, 1979

I have been looking inward at beliefs I hold that hinder clear vision: 1) I believe in *effort*, that things have to be *worked for* or are not worth achieving (fairly typical of our American Puritan heritage), thus I find it difficult to hold the belief that vision is effortless. *I* have to do it; I have to *try*. 2) I like to achieve as a result of the preceding belief, and also like to achieve what is *difficult*. So I make seeing difficult so that, later, I can say, "That sure was hard, but I did it."

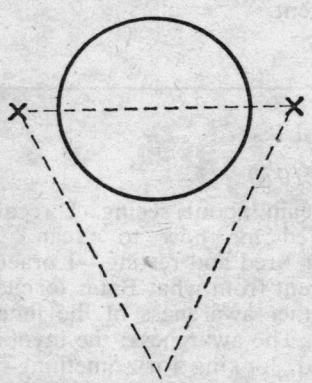

swing from left to right

Close your eyes and hold up your right hand again. Now point your nose to the tops of your fingers. Where is your hand? Yes, it is below your nose. Now point your nose at the bottom of your hand, and you will see how your hand seems to be above where you are pointing. Proceed to look above and below your hand, first with eyes both closed, then with them open. Then do the same thing with the chart, looking above and below it. See the diagrams below.

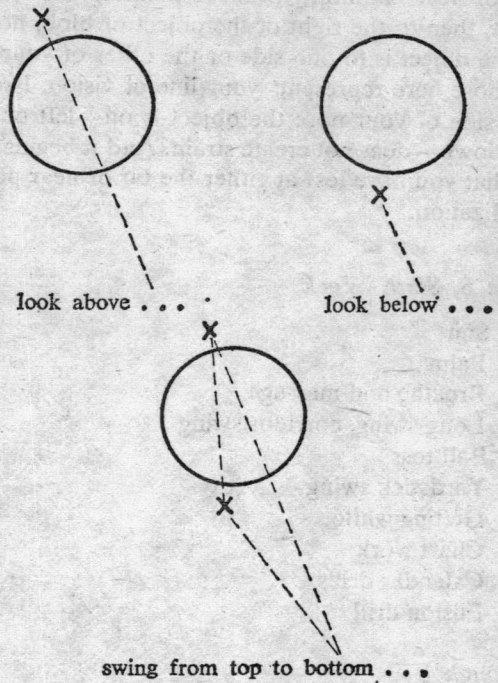

look above . . .

look below . . .

swing from top to bottom . . .

When you look at the bottom of any object, it will appear to be above your line of vision; when you look at the top, the object will appear to be below your line of vision. This awareness will help you to recognize the very real movement that occurs with vision.

Always do the relaxation exercises—sunning, palming, massaging, the long swing and ball toss before you do the yardstick swing or the chart work.

Integrate what you have learned in the chart work in the following ways. Pick an object at any distance from you. It does not matter whether you can "see" it, or even recognize it as long as it is a blob of something out there, or near in. Simply practice pointing your nose to the left, then to the right of the object or blob, noticing how the object is to one side or the other of your nose. Your nose here represents your line of vision. Noticing which side of your nose the object is on—left or right, up or down—does not create strain. And it begins to get you what you have lost at either the far or near point—centralization.

Lesson 6, Sixth Week

1. Sun
2. Palm
3. Breathe and massage
4. Long swing, corridor swing
5. Ball toss
6. Yardstick swing
7. Getting white
8. Chart work
9. Calendar drills
10. Fusion drill

1 through 8

Do all of these exercises as before.

8. Calendar Drill

If, after the chart work, you feel some tension, do a little palming and massage before going on to this exercise. The calendar drill can also be alternated with the chart work so that one day you do the one, the next day, the other. You should obtain a large calendar page with big black numbers against a white background, together with a very small calendar of the same month and year, which you can mount on a popsicle stick or tongue depressor, so that it can be held very close to your face. Often, a calendar will contain in the corners these smaller calendars of the months preceding and following. You can also have a third, medium-sized calendar of the same month and year, so that you can have three, rather than only two, distances with which to work.

Place the large calendar at a comfortable distance. Hold the small, mounted calendar in front of you, also at a comfortable distance.

If you are nearsighted, start the exercise with the small calendar near you. If you are farsighted, start it with the large calendar in the distance.

Close your eyes. Imagine your calendar in front of you (near or far). Point your nose to the left side, and notice how the calendar is to the right of your line of vision. Swing to the right side and notice how it is now to the left. Continue this exercise in exactly the same way you do the chart work. Swing the calendar, near and far, small and large, first with your eyes closed, then with them open. Remember to blink and breathe.

9. Fusion Drill

Take a length of string about 18 inches long, and string a brightly colored bead in its middle, tying a knot on either side of the bead so that it stays centered.

Hold the string with the bead taut between your two hands, directly out in front of your nose, as illustrated. Aim your nose at the point on the string where your thumb locks it against your index finger. (If you are farsighted, you may have to hold the string farther away—you may hold it as close as two to three inches, or as far as eight to ten). Now point your nose along the string to the bead. Blink. Breathe.

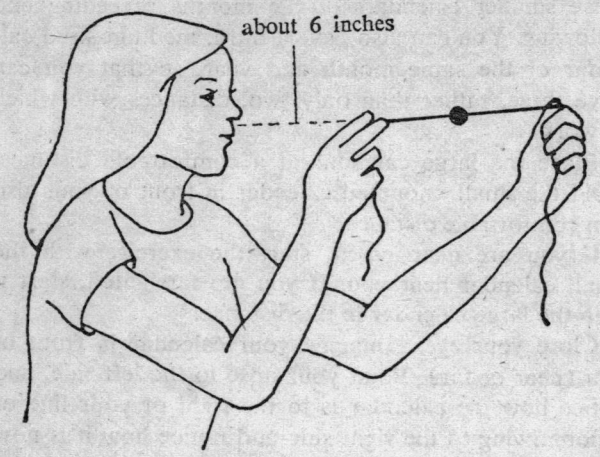

Now aim your nose out to the point where the thumb of your other hand holds it. What happens to the string as you point at these three different points?

When you aim at the nearest point, the rest of the string appears to open out into a *V* shape.

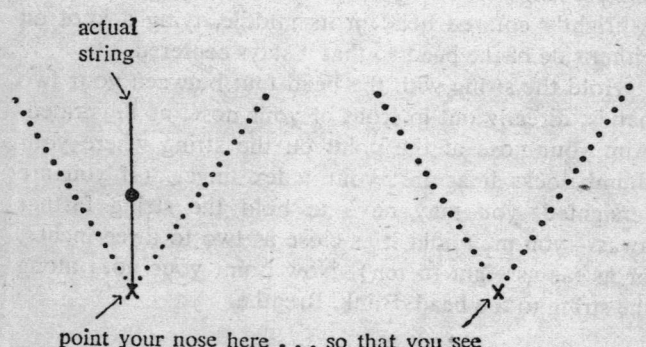

point your nose here . . . so that you see

When you point your nose at the bead, you notice an X.

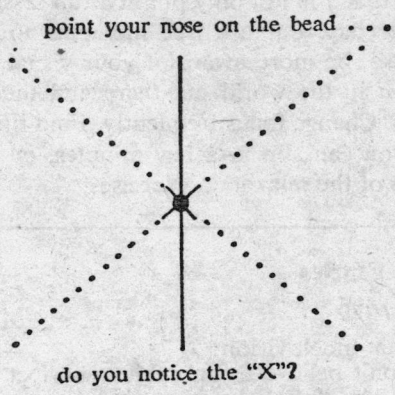

And when you point to the far point, you get an A without the crossbar.

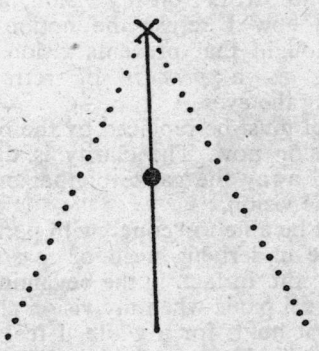

Be sure to blink and breathe and move your nose. If you do not get the A-V-X shapes, relax and practice. If you still do not get them after a week, then read the material in the next chapter under the heading "Squint."

Continue to integrate the various exercises into your daily life so that you not only put in a full session of the exercises per day, but use free moments to get extra practice. Also, be more aware of your visual curiosity. Be *interested* in the world out there and the world in close to you. Change focus frequently. Find times of the day when you can slip in a few minutes, or even seconds, of one of the relaxation exercises.

Journal Entries

July 22, 1979

Beliefs that block vision:

1. I don't believe I can achieve perfect vision. My eyes are "weak," and seeing occurs in the eyes.

This must be replaced by the belief that it is the *mind* that does the seeing. It is the thought that I can't see that prevents the seeing.

2. I have to "work" on my vision, which illustrates again how I refuse the notion that it is merely a thought that prevents vision. I see the whole thing as a *process* of retraining and strengthening the *eyes*.

This belief must be replaced by the belief that I have my vision now. The clarity is there; I but need to pull away the gauze of that one thought that blurs the vision.

3. I won't be able to "cope" with perfect vision. I have some underlying need or reason to have imperfect vision. In fact, in the beginning, I would experience real panic when my vision cleared, and lately when it holds for a while, I feel a discomfort inside, a kind of questioning, like what am I supposed to do with what I see out there? I somehow feel as though I am responsible for doing something with what I see, hence I feel a bit overwhelmed when it's all crisp and clear.

> This must be replaced by the realization that I no longer have whatever need there might have originally been, hence there is nothing to "cope" with! I simply have a habit that has already been altered to such an extent that all that needs to be changed now is that negative thought.
>
> 4. I need *time* to get used to seeing clearly.
>
> To be replaced by the realization that I've had plenty of time. Now I am *ready*.

Lesson 7, Seventh Week

1. Sun
2. Palm
3. Breathe and massage
4. Long swing, corridor swing
5. Edging
6. Ball toss
7. Getting white
8. Chart work or calendar work
9. Massage
10. Fusion

1 through 3

Sun, palm and massage as usual.

4. Long Swing

Obtain a piece of sturdy but bendable wire, and cut it so that it is about 29 inches long. TV wire, available in hardware stores, is perfect. Bend the wire as follows to make what is called the Bates Gate:

1. Bend the first three to four inches of wire to form a shallow arch. (See illustration.) This will rest across the top of your head, from the middle of your scalp to just above your ear.

Step 1

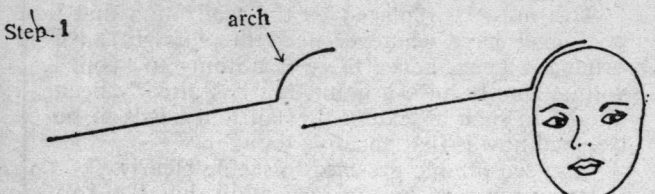

2. Bend the remainder of the wire back around your head to form a circle, similar to a hat band, all the way to the front. Stop the circle in the middle of your forehead.

Step 2

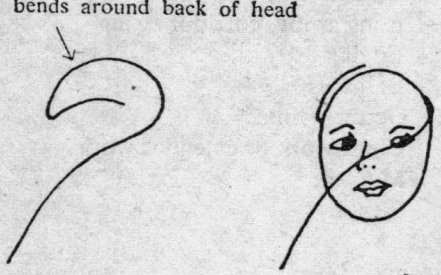

3. Now bend the remainder of the wire straight out from the center of your forehead.

Step 3

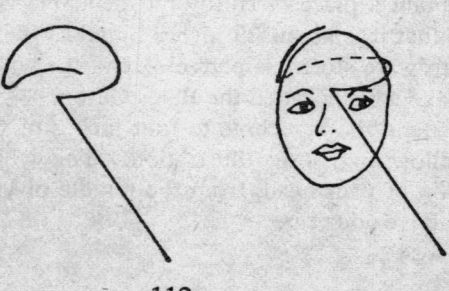

4. Bend the last few inches of wire straight down about three inches directly in front of your nose. What you want is a portion of wire out in front of your nose to form the "gate" described below.

Step 4

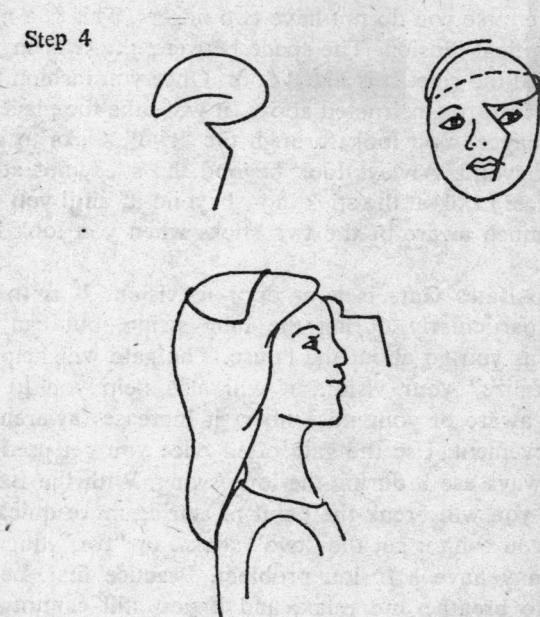

You have two eyes, each with its own retina, which receives an image, just as the film of a camera receives an image. But when you look at an object, you see not two, but one. Why? The mind puts the two images from the eyes together to form one. This process is called fusion—i.e., the mind fuses together the two separate images.

Hold your index finger up straight and touch your nose. Now move your finger straight out directly in front of your nose, about six inches away. Look at the finger. You see one finger. Now look beyond the finger to a distant object straight out in front of you. While seeing the flower, or table—whatever object you have chosen to see—it will seem as if you have two fingers in front of you.

Of course you do not have two fingers. This is a normal optical illusion. The space between the two fingers is called the gate. It is like a door. Once you fashion the Bates Gate, as instructed above, it will take the place of your finger. You look through the "two" sticks to objects beyond. Always look beyond the stick, not at it. Practice. Look at the stick, now beyond it, until you are very much aware of the two sticks when you look beyond.

The Bates Gate is your door to vision. It is to be used particularly during the long swing, but can be worn as you go about the house. The gate will help to "centralize" your vision; it will also help you to be more aware of your nose fiber; it increases awareness of movement. Use the gate often once you get used to it. Always use it during the long swing. With the Bates Gate, you will break the habit of staring more quickly.

If you cannot get the "two" sticks, or "two" fingers, you may have a fusion problem. Practice first, being sure to breathe and relax, and if you still cannot get "two," go to the section in the next chapter called "Squint."

To use the Bates Gate during the long swing, you will have to slow down a bit, because the sensation of movement is much greater with the gate on. Just let the world come in to you through the gate. Let everything go by in the opposite direction. If the gate bothers you at first, remove it, but keep practicing with it, even if only for short periods. It is a great aid to vision.

Lesson 8, Eighth Week

1 through 10

Sun, palm, massage, long swing, corridor swing, ball toss, yardstick swing, massage, fusion exercise, palm.

11. Chart Work

You have worked with your chart for two weeks now. It should swing from side to side and up and down for you with relative ease. If it does not, then skip this and the next exercise until the swinging takes place easily. Unless the swinging of the chart and calendars comes easily, the next exercises will only produce strain.

Rather than swing the whole chart now, you will move your nose to the left edge of the first letter or letters on the chart, noticing how the letter or letters are to the right of your line of vision. Now swing to the right and notice how the letter or letters are to the left. Swing the next whole row of letters, then the next, down the chart as far down as the swinging comes easily to you.

If the rows swing easily, practice swinging individual letters, the large ones first, then down to the smaller ones. Swinging the letters, both from side to side and up and down, may take several weeks or months of practice. *Take your time*. Remember the rule: blink, breathe, swing your nose. Your vision will improve as you are able to swing small things both close up and in the distance. Work at whatever distance is *comfortable* for you.

> **Journal Entry**
>
> *January 20, 1980*
>
> Vision coming along nicely. In my sunning, I'm working on letting the white light, about which I read more in the visualization book (*Seeing With the Mind's Eye*), drop down my body through my eyes, entering, soothing, warming, or cooling—whatever the various parts of my body need. Lastly, I'm suggesting that it rest my mind, allowing it to permit and accept vision. It's coming more and more, holding longer, coming when I least expect it, when I'm not *doing* anything about it. I know now that the day will come when I will scarcely be able to imagine myself as a person who could not see clearly before. The mind is an incredible power; it works with or without our conscious control. It can be compared to a computer in a way—*it* is the program; I have to become the programmer on a conscious level; otherwise, I program my mind willy-nilly and am at the mercy of any and all of the negative and positive influences in my life. In terms of vision, the program has for years been a negative one. Now it's time to change.

12. Calendar Work

Do the same exercises as above, with both the small and large calendars, using the numbers in place of the letters. These two exercises can be alternated, or you may prefer one to the other. Do whichever comes easiest to you.

By now, you will have your "favorites" among the exercises. Do most frequently, and for the longest time, those that make you feel the best—the best meaning the most relaxed.

Lesson 9, Ninth Week

This lesson begins the reading exercises. From this point on, do your regular routine, including whatever exercises you enjoy most, but being sure to include sunning, palming, massaging and the long swing.

Reading Step 1: Flashing

Cover your left eye with your palm, leaving both eyes open. Point your nose straight ahead. Hold your right hand out, the palm toward you, as far in front of you as your arm extends. Hold your hand over to the left side of your nose, and look at it with your open eye. Quickly bring the palm of your extended hand up to your open eye, then extend your arm out again so that you "scissors" your hand in and out rapidly. At the same time, blink rapidly. Do this ten times. Now cover the other eye and do the exercise exactly the same way, but on the opposite side.

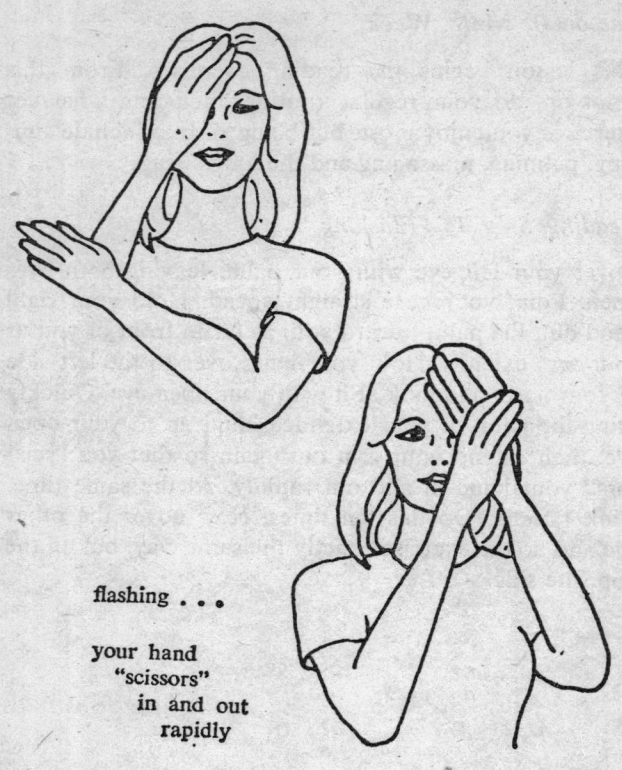

flashing . . .

your hand
"scissors"
in and out
rapidly

Reading Step 2: Getting White

Do the getting-white exercise here (see Lesson 4).

Reading Step 3: Reading Card

Cut out the reading page at the very front of the book, entitled Fundamentals of Eye Training and hold it about 12 inches in front of you. If the letters are blurred, relax—you are only to see *white*, and you can see that well at any distance. Now point your nose at the top edge of the page and edge it several times, blinking and breathing. Be sure you have good light. You may want to use your sunning lamp to shine directly on the paper. As you edge the page, do you notice a white line along the edge? Be sure to tell yourself to edge the *paper* side of the page, not the *air* side. If you do not get a white line or white glow on the edge, take a deep breath, close your eyes, and imagine one as you now edge the page with your eyes closed. Take your time and, farsighted people, be particularly sensitive to yourselves. If you notice tension, pause, and palm or sun or massage before you continue. This week, just practice this edging with the page at the 12-inch reading distance. Do a lot of imagining the nearness of the page with your eyes closed. Pay no attention to the letters. Then, opening your eyes, point your nose to the left side of the paper, noticing how the page is on the right side of your nose. Swing the paper both sideways and up and down, just as you do with both the chart and the calendars.

Lesson 10, Tenth Week

Continue all steps as before and do the first three steps of the reading exercise.

Reading Step 4

Holding toward you the side of the page with the letters on it, point your nose to the left side of the big *C* on the first line. Now slowly circle *in the white* around the *C*. Do this with your nose, and blink and breathe. You will notice that the *C* seems to have a halo of light around it, a white glow. If you do not perceive the glow, close your eyes and imagine it, telling yourself that it is there. Make no effort to force it. Gradually the glow will come. Open your eyes and circle the *A*, again in the white. Close your eyes, and imagine the white around the *A*. Let the white background be the positive, the letter the negative. Remember, it takes no effort to perceive white. Check that you are holding the paper at the proper reading distance—approximately 12 inches.

Continue circling the letters or, for variety, swing them from side to side and up and down, as with your chart and calendar exercises, always staying in the white. Breathe and blink. Close your eyes and imagine the movement, then open and swing something in the distance. Circle as many letters as you wish, as far down the page as is comfortable. Be on guard against squinting or holding your head at an unnatural angle. Point your nose at the letter you are circling, and let your attention follow where your nose fiber touches.

Reading Step 5: Painting the Arc

Put the page down, and close your eyes. Imagine you are painting an arc on the floor or table in front of you. Imagine you have a paintbrush on the end of your nose, a magic brush that can change colors at a thought from you. Choose your colors so that they are vivid in your mind. Use such terms as *sky blue,* or *cornflower blue,* or *indigo blue*, rather than the vaguer term of simply *blue*. Change colors frequently, and do the exercise for as long as you wish.

Lesson 11, Eleventh Week

Do your usual routine and all the reading steps.

Reading Step 6: Reading the Page

Turn the page to the reading lesson side. Edge the page again, noticing the white line. Now point your nose in the white just at the bottom of the letters in the first line of the title. You might wish to use a white card, such as the back of an index card, to cover the print below in order to help you to keep your attention in the space *between* the lines of print.

Draw a line with your nose just under the letters. Pay no attention to the letters—you are simply drawing a white line with your nose under the print. Let the letters come in to you, but make no effort to go after them. Fairly quickly—at least faster than you normally read—paint the white line under each line of print several times, and move on down the page as long as you are comfortable. Close and imagine the line sometimes. Occasionally look off across the room or out the window. Be aware of your blinking and breathing. *Make no effort*. With relaxation and practice in thinking white, and reading in the white, the print will be clear.

REMEMBER: The print on the page is perfectly distinct and perfectly black. The blurring is in your mind because you are straining to see. Relax. The print is waiting for you to see it.

Seeing is not looking, as hearing is not listening.

In general, read by quickly painting a white line just under the print. When your mind/eyes lose their sluggishness at the near point, their natural movement will be rapid enough to take in the print with no effort whatsoever. When you finish the bottom of a page or column, as in a newspaper or magazine, rest your eyes by simply closing them briefly, then looking off and swinging on an object in the distance. As you paint the line, the whole book, or page, will appear to move slightly from side to side. Remember to stop if you feel you are becoming tense; palm or massage before you go on. *Always* do the relaxation exercises before you ever try your reading exercise.

Middle-Age Sight

Some people, as they age, lose the flexibility of the lens inside the eye; this condition usually develops in the forties and fifties. For the purposes of these exercises, people with this problem should assume they are farsighted and follow the program as the farsighted person is directed to do. Apparently the relaxation of the muscles that accompanies the Bates exercises helps to *compensate* for the less flexible lens, thus allowing better vision to occur. The shorter the time period that the lesser vision has existed, the faster the improvement of the vision.

Lesson 12, Twelfth Week

Any of the following variations may be added, or substituted for the exercises given in the first 11 lessons.

Sunning

a. Imagine that the light enters through your closed lids, fills the inside of your head, then slowly begins to sink down your neck to your shoulders, and then down your whole body, slowly sinking, bringing warmth and relaxation wherever it reaches. Imagine it moves in the way that warm honey would move. Feel it sinking, opening your lungs, softening every muscle. Follow its course down to your toes.

b. Imagine that you breathe in the colors of the light spectrum. Make no change in your breathing, first simply notice your inhaling. Each time you inhale, the red of a rainbow fills your head. At first it is like a mist, but as you continue to breathe, it gradually intensifies until your whole head is filled with that red. Then let it out on your breath, paying attention now to your exhaling until the color is gone. Now breathe in the orange in the same way, and let it out after it has reached its highest point of intensity. Breathe in the yellow, green, blue, and purple in the same way, one after another. Then imaginitively mix all the colors together to make a very bright white light, and breathe that in and out in the same way.

Palming

a. Lie or sit in your palming posture and simply listen to your favorite *soothing* music.

b. Palm without visualizing. Simply allow whatever sounds are around you to come in to you. Notice how you hear without effort, how your sense of hearing slips from one sound to another without clinging to the last sound, without *staring* at it, so to speak. You hear without any effort. This is the way seeing also occurs.

Mental Drills

During your work or school day, you can take a few moments to relax by doing any one of the following mental drills. Because the mind can think of only one thing at any one time, and because these activities are based on a rhythmic rocking motion, your careful concentration on one of these mental drills will produce relaxation even in the midst of the busiest days. You should do any of these exercises with your eyes loosely closed, or while palming, if that is convenient.

1. Swing the O With your eyes closed, use your nose fiber to paint a black *O* on a white background in your imagination. Put a black dot on either side of the *O*, as illustrated. Now, point your nose to the left dot and swing across the white central space to the other, swinging back and forth from side to side until the *O* seems to slip past in the direction opposite to the one in which you are swinging.

Put dots now at the top and bottom of the *O*, and swing vertically. The *O* will seem to move up and down opposite to you. If the illusion of motion does not come easily, go back to the exercise with your own hand held in front of your face, as described in Lesson 5. And breathe and relax. The movement, after all, is only an illusion.

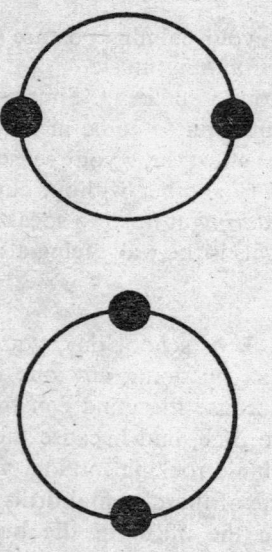

Swing the O

2. Swing the triangle In your imagination draw a black triangle with equal sides, as illustrated. On either side of the triangle's base, place a black dot. Breathe deeply, point your nose to the left black dot, and swing across to the other dot. As you swing from dot to dot, the triangle will seem to slip past in the opposite direction. Now draw another triangle, one that is inverted, and place dots on either side of its tip. Again, swing your nose from dot to dot and simply note how the triangle slips up and down in the direction opposite to your movement. You need pay no attention to the triangle. Just slide your nose up and down from dot to dot.

3. Swing the bars Imagine that you have in front of you a large piece of white paper upon which a heavy black horizontal line, or bar, has been drawn. There is a dot at either end of the bar. As with the triangle and *O*, swing from dot to dot, noticing how the bar shifts back and forth opposite to you. Imagine that the bar is vertical now, with dots at top and bottom, and swing up and down. Then imagine the bar in one, then the other, diagonal, as with the yardstick swing, and swing your nose from dot to dot along those planes.

4. Swing the domino Everyone, at some time or another, has played with dominoes. Imagine that you are now holding one in your hand. Feel its smooth front, with the raised ridge that divides the domino in half. Feel also the indentation the two white dots each make. Now, in your imagination, look at the domino. One very white dot is in the center of the smooth, very black upper half of the domino. Another is in the center of the bottom half. Hold the domino horizontally at a comfortable distance. (Even in your imagination, certain distances will be comfortable, others not.) Point your nose first at one dot, then at the other, swinging back and forth between the two. Notice how the whole domino seems to move back and forth in the direction opposite to your movement.

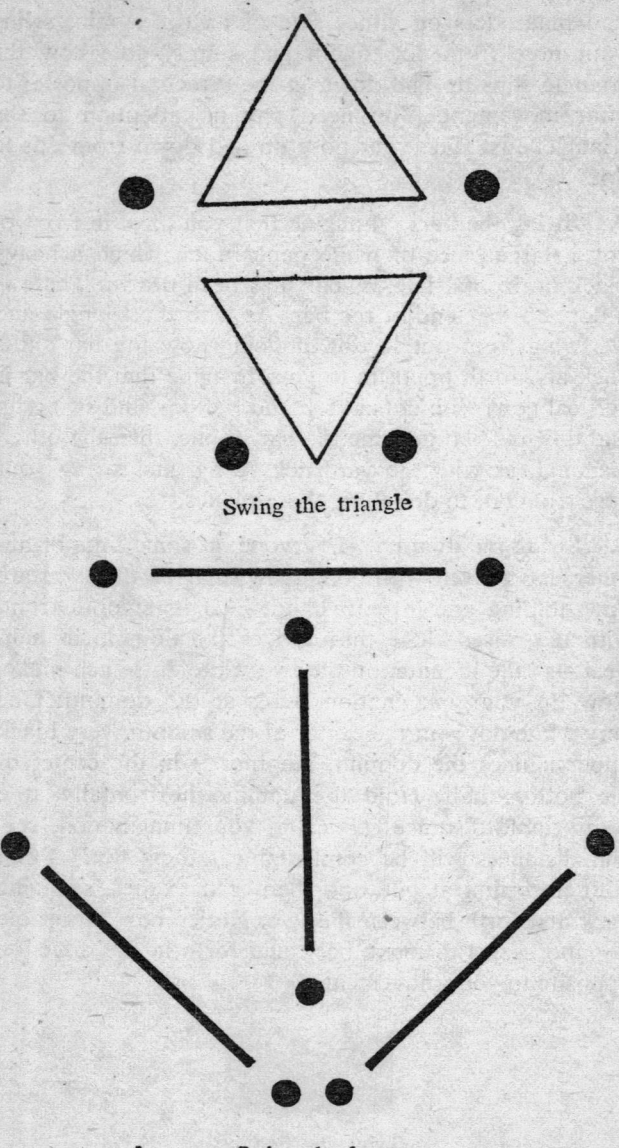

Now hold the domino vertically, and swing from dot to dot as above. The domino will appear to move up and down opposite to your movement.

5. Swing the owl Besides geometric figures, as with the preceding exercises, you can use just about any object to lull your mind into a state of rest. Movement is the key, movement that is easy and rocking and opposite to your head's movements. So now, imagine an owl—or any bird for that matter, one you can easily envision—sitting in the center of a crescent moon, the points of which are turned upward, as in the illustration. Now run your nose up to one point of the moon and let it drop along the curve up to the other point. Swing back and forth in an easy motion, and notice how the owl seems to rock back and forth, almost as if it were in a cradle.

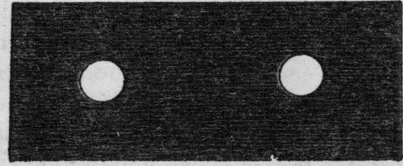

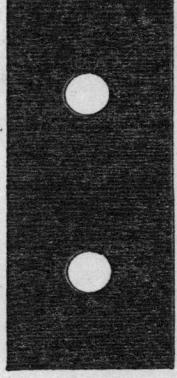

Swing the domino

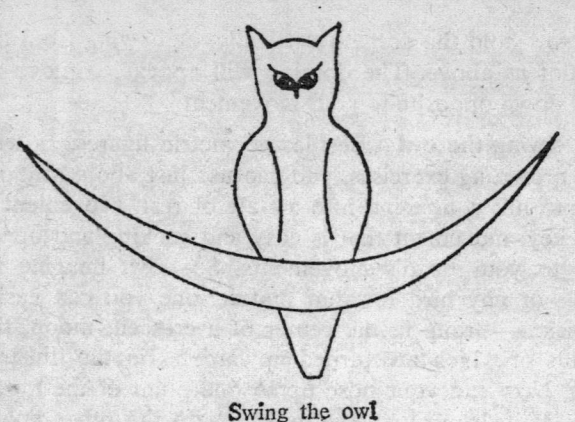

Swing the owl

6. Swing the scales Imagine a pair of old-fashioned jeweler's scales like the ones illustrated. Then point your nose at the left tray and run it smoothly up the center chain to the balancing bar, across the balancing bar, and down the center chain of the right tray, down into the tray. Reverse, and repeat going from one tray up across the balancing bar and down to the other tray. As you do this, the tray in which you put your nose will seem to move downward and the one on the other side upward, almost as if your attention had its own weight.

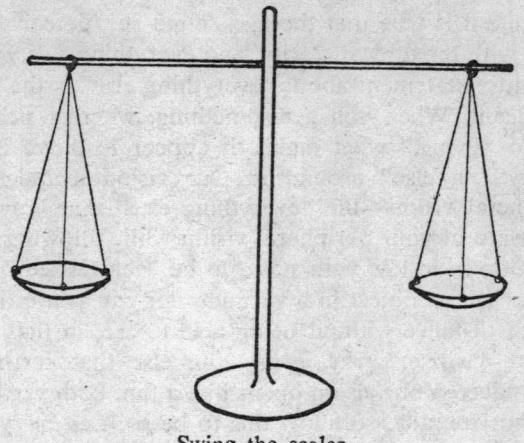

Swing the scales

Ball Toss

Play ball in your imagination, pretending to throw the ball way out over the ocean so that it gets tinier and tinier. Then follow it as it comes back to you from that great distance, watching it get larger and brighter as it comes closer, right up to your nose. And whenever you really play any kind of ball games, keep your *nose* on the ball.

Centralization

You have several exercises in which you "swing" things. Notice how when you point your nose to the left side of any object, the right side is "worse"—that is, you don't see the right side as well as you see the left side, where your attention is focused. You do *not* see the left side *better*—that creates *strain*. It takes no effort to see something worse, so tell yourself: *The other side is worse*. And notice how this is true. Point from side to side and up and down at near and far distances, noticing how the other side is worse.

While it is true that the eyes/mind see/perceive one point with the utmost clarity, and everything else worse, this latter statement about "everything else" is the most significant. When you get something, whether near or far, to "swing," what makes it appear to move is the "everything else" around it. Our vision includes the peripheral vision—the "everything else" that is worse. Be aware of your peripheral vision while allowing your attention to follow your nose, to be "centralized." You cannot see an object in a vacuum, nor can you estimate size or distance without being able to see, in that peripheral, "worse," way, everything else that surrounds that object. Your vision opens like a fan, both vertically and horizontally, so allow this to be so. *Let everything come in to you.*

Fusion

Gradually, as you work with the *A-V-X* string, lengthen the string. Tie it to a piece of furniture, and string several beads on it, practicing along the length of the string at the various points. Nearsighted people should work toward the distance, farsighted toward the nose.

Reading

Gradually read in the smaller print, and when you can comfortably read the smallest print on your page at 12 inches, begin to read that print closer and closer to your nose until you can read it with ease at three to four inches from your nose. Remember always to "read" the white line, not the print.

Summary

Finally, and perhaps most of all, watch your own attitudes and beliefs. If you sincerely believe that you *can-*

not and *will not* improve your vision, then you most likely will not. You have to put your thinking behind your actions. Just as sometime in the past you began to *think* that your vision was poor, and lo and behold your vision became poor, now you must reverse that thought and replace it with a new one:

I see perfectly clearly with the greatest of ease.

And be sensitive to yourself. Recognize tension when it exists and do something about it.

Journal Entry

March 6, 1980

Vision: my long swing is smoother now, though I still block out parts of the field as I turn. But I remember how it used to be, whole sections of it simply not perceived. I also feel inwardly surer, much less afraid of not being able to see and much more aware of how that *is* the problem for me: I am (or have been) afraid that I won't see, so I fulfill that inner expectation constantly. When I do relax, I see: it's that simple. I am then able to let go, and my eyes focus on the object, no matter what the distance, with ease.

CHAPTER 8

For more serious disorders: Ambliopia and squint, cataracts, detached retina, glaucoma, night blindness

While the Bates work, done correctly, cannot hurt anyone, if you have more serious vision disorders, it is important, for your own protection, to get an ophthalmologist's approval for doing the exercises. It is also important that you truly *relax*. People with serious vision problems are tense people, sometimes in pain, and relaxation may not come easily. Only you can tell if a specific exercise is causing more, or less, tension; if it causes more, then stop. Without relaxation, the exercises are of no benefit whatever. You must also be more patient than someone with simple myopia, hyperopia, or astigmatism. Results often come slowly, in tiny increments, not dramatically. But with patience, they can and do come. It might be worth your time and money to travel to a Bates teacher occasionally, so that you can be sure you are doing the exercises correctly. A teacher near you can be located by contacting the Bates-Corbett Teachers' Association at 11303 Meadow View Road, El Cajon, California 92020.

Ambliopia and Squint

Squint is a condition in which one or both eyes turn off focus. The eye or eyes may turn inward toward the nose (called convergent squint), or outward (divergent squint), or even up or down (vertical squint). In any case, since each eye views something different from the other, the result is double vision, a phenomenon that the mind cannot tolerate. Thus, what happens is that the *mind* turns off on one side so that only one eye, and one side of the brain, does the seeing. The turning-off of one side of the vision is called "ambliopia," often called "lazy eye." The ambliopic eye is neither diseased nor shows refractive error, but its nerves are numb from disuse. The condition of squint affects the whole physical, mental, and emotional state of being. Most sufferers are highly nervous, and usually very intelligent.

There are basically two aims in working with squint. The first is to stimulate the lazy eye, to awaken that part of the brain once again; the second is to work toward straightening the wayward eye or eyes so that fusion occurs. Underlying both of these aims is the need for relaxation because only with relaxation can progress be made.

If you are a parent of a squint child, please read the chapter on working with children before you embark on any program to help your child. Unfortunately, parents often make the worst teachers because they want success for the little one too desperately. The child responds with a bad case of nerves and often grows worse.

To achieve fusion in squint takes a great deal of patience both on the teacher's and the student's part. It can indeed be very frustrating, and the student needs all the support and understanding he or she can get. The student also needs to maintain relaxation, a nearly impossible feat with an anxious parent hovering over him or her. Then, when fusion begins to occur, it often happens that the impact is very nearly overwhelming. The person may feel dizzy, faint, or nauseated—situations that have to be handled calmly. And though these symptoms pass fairly soon, the child may not want to achieve fusion, in order to avoid the unpleasantness. He or she must be coaxed into working toward fusion. Such a time is hard enough on a somewhat disinterested friend or teacher, but for a parent it can be extremely trying. So please do yourself and your child a favor: read the chapter following this one.

If you yourself have squint or ambliopia, however, read on. Be aware that it will perhaps be months before any improvement shows up. Also be aware that your first goal is relaxation. And if one or both of your eyes have already been operated upon, then you will have even greater difficulty because the operated eye might be too tight to achieve shifting, the normal rapid movement that occurs in naturally relaxed eyes.

For your program, follow the lessons as outlined in the preceding chapter, adding the exercises listed below.

Lesson 1, First Week

First off, you must obtain an eye patch made of soft black fabric that closes off the light entirely, but places no pressure on the eye itself.

1. Massage and breathe as described in Chapter 6.
2. Sun, but sun often for two to three minutes five or six times a day. Start your sunning with the patch on your stronger eye, then remove it, and sun both eyes together for the same amount of time that you sunned with the patch on. In cases of alternate squint, in which only one, but either, eye is used at a time, patch one eye, then the other, and leave the patch on only for short periods.
3. Palm, but palm for ten minutes ten times a day.
4. Easy open, easy close.

5. Blinking.

6. Finger swing. In addition to the above, do this swing often throughout the day. Use your patch—always on the stronger eye—for half the time you do this, and palm briefly after you have patched your eye, in order to allow both eyes to coordinate in the light.

Hold your index finger straight up, about six inches in front of your nose. Slowly swing your head from side to side, letting your gaze go out into the distance. Your finger will seem to move from side to side in a direction opposite to the one in which you are moving your head. Be sure to blink and breathe.

7. Head Posture. Squint sufferers tilt their heads to offset their disability. Have someone help you here by observing the position of your head until you get it straight. Then practice often to learn what it feels like when your head is held correctly. This will be bothersome because, in straightening your head, you initially will lose some vision. Keep at it. The position of your head is the first step.

Lesson 2, Second Week

Follow this lesson as outlined in the previous chapter, except use the patch as directed for Lesson 1, and add the patch while doing the long swing and the ball toss. Remember to use the patch for only half the exercises; then, for the other half, do them with both eyes unpatched. And *always* palm briefly after you have patched. You should also do the finger swing and continue working on your head posture.

And, for this lesson, and all that follow, just briefly attempt this simple fusion exercise. Hold your index finger in front of your nose, as in the finger swing, but do not swing your head. Simply point your nose at an object *beyond* your finger, as, for example, a chair on the opposite side of the room, or a bush or tree or house, if you are outdoors. Do you have two fingers? Do not look at your finger because then you will have only one; look beyond it into the distance, and the finger will appear to break into two. If this happens, then you are achieving fusion; if not, *do not* make any effort; just check and let it go. The most important thing you are doing is a) relaxing, and b) getting the retina of your weaker eye and the side of the mind behind that eye to wake up. Until that happens, fusion will not occur.

Lesson 3, Third Week

Continue as before; add the corridor swing, using the patch, and patch for the conversation swing as well.

If you do not know whether your eye/eyes go in or out, find out from your doctor so that you can now begin to work on your phoria. *Phoria* means the tendency of your line of vision to turn inward, outward, up, or down. For two weeks now, you have been "awakening" your weaker eye. You must continue to do this for as long as necessary. Be patient; it may take time. But now you can also begin to work on straightening the turned eye. Do the following exercise.

Inward-Turning Eye/Eyes

Point your nose straight ahead. Patch your straight, or stronger, eye. Using the arm on the same side as your weaker eye, raise the arm, pointing your index finger toward the ceiling. Then slowly lower it, all the while following your finger with your nose (which should be pointed straight ahead, not at the finger), moving up and down, and your weaker eye. Keep raising and lowering the arm and following it. Be sure to blink and breathe. Because you are moving your arm off to the side, your weaker eye must turn outward in order to follow your pointed finger. It is your *eye* that turns in this exercise, *not* your head.

Outward-Turning Eye/Eyes

Follow the directions for the preceding exercise, only raise and lower your arm on the other side of your body so that your outward-turning eye is pulled inward toward your nose.

Eye/Eyes with Vertical Squint

If your eye pulls downward, swing your arm above your head in a horizontal line, so the eye must look upward. Do the exact opposite, i.e., swing your arm below your nose, if your eye or eyes pull upward.

With alternate squint, be sure to work both eyes in the direction opposite to your phoria.

Lesson 4 and Following

You may proceed with the lessons in Chapter 6 exactly as they are outlined there with these exceptions and additions.

Lesson 4

Never use the patch while driving. Add the following swing.

High Hat Swing Hold up your hands, palms up and facing out in front of you, at shoulder level. Then swing your head from side to side. Your upheld hands will appear to move in the direction opposite to your movement. Do this with and without your patch.

Lesson 5

Use the patch with the yardstick swing and with chart work.

Continue doing all the swings and exercises described above for as long as necessary until your weaker eye has significantly improved in picking up vision, and until you begin to achieve fusion. Then go on to Lesson 6 and follow the rest of the lessons as anyone else would. Continue, however, working with your patch, with lots of short periods of sunning and palming, and lots of *brief* activity with the *A-V-X* string. Be sure you are thoroughly relaxed when you do the fusion drill or work with the halo.

Cataracts

Cataract is a condition in which sediment is deposited in the lens of the eye, creating an opacity there that clouds the vision. Dr. Bates believed that cataracts were caused mainly by tension and staring. Thus, the relaxation exercises—particularly the massage and palming and the various swings—are most important. In addition, you must find ways to deal with the tension in your life, and to avoid dwelling on negative thoughts and problems. Talk and think about *pleasant* memories. Circulation in the lens is critical in treating cataracts, so foods and supplements that aid good circulation and that purify the blood are most helpful. You should also get exercise and fresh air. Do lots of breathing exercises, and always watch your breathing because it is an indication of the degree of tension or relaxation.

At first, stick with the first four lessons in Chapter 6. Palm a lot and often, and always palm twice as long as you sun. When you sun, be aware of your light sensitivity. Sun indoors with a low-wattage incandescent light bulb, or outdoors in the shade for as many weeks or months as you need to in order to gradually get used to the light. Blinking will be difficult for you. Practice it often, and close your eyes and rest them a lot. Do a lot of memory and imagination exercises with your eyes closed.

Always use your eyes at only the distances that are *easy* for you. Walk up to things if necessary, and swing your nose around everything so that you do not stare. Do the long swing frequently as well as the finger swing as described in the section on ambliopia and squint, Lesson 1, Number 6.

When sunning is easy for you, your breathing easy and relaxed, and, in general, you feel an overall improvement in terms of relaxation, then start Lesson 5 and work on through the 12 lessons. But take your time. You might do the first four lessons over a period of months, then add one lesson every few weeks. Do not be discouraged or impatient. Speed is not nature's way, nor should it be your aim. Have your cataracts checked every few months, or as often as your doctor recommends.

Detached Retina

Relaxation of the mind is necessary in cases involving detached retina. To accomplish this, you must have a great deal of rest, and palming flat on your back is the best way to achieve it. Frequent periods of palming, *so long as you do not get bored or restless*, together with short periods of sunning—*nothing more*—are the proper course of action until the retina has reattached. During this period and afterward, avoid quick, nervous movements, and *never* bend over. Bend from the knees if such a movement is necessary. Do not strain to see.

Sun in a reclining position, and move your head slowly and easily. Listen to music or the radio, or have someone read to you while you palm. It takes weeks for the eye to heal. Once it has—i.e., if you have not opted for surgery—you may start, *very gently*, doing the other exercises outlined in the preceding chapter, if you need to improve your overall vision. Do the exercises for short periods, very easily, and rest often with palming. Keep in close contact with your doctor on your progress.

Glaucoma

Glaucoma may be painless or painful, depending on various circumstances. In either case it is a dangerous eye disorder because it can lead to blindness if left untreated. Bates helped many sufferers of glaucoma because relaxation is essential in alleviating both the symptoms and the disease.

Sun often and for short periods. If you have difficulty visualizing, then let that go, but keep your head moving in various swings—horizontal, vertical, circular.

Palm a lot. Use the radio or music if you have trouble remembering. Have a friend read to you while you palm. As the symptoms lessen in intensity, your memory and imagination will improve.

Work for ease and clarity of vision at whatever distance is easy for you. Do not work for distance until the glaucoma has cleared up, because this will induce strain, which is what is giving you the problem to begin with.

Paste white adhesive on black paper and swing on these in place of the calendars and chart in the regular program.

Do 200 long swings at night before going to bed. Avoid tiring your eyes and rest often.

Finally, do these mental relaxation drills. Remember, your mind can only handle one thing at a time. It does this with such lightning rapidity, however, that it *appears* as if many things are going on at once, so when you are completely engrossed in one of these mental drills, you will not experience pain.

1. Swing the O

Imagine a black letter *O* on a piece of white paper. Point your nose to the left side of the O, then slide across it and point to the right. The O will begin to swing as you do, seeming to move in a direction opposite to yours. Do this a number of times, then swing from the top of the O to the bottom in the same way. Notice how the O seems to move up and down in the opposite direction to your movement.

2. Swing the bar

Imagine a bar, black and solid on a white background. Swing it horizontally as you did with the O, then stand the bar upright and swing up and down. Again, notice the oppositional movement.

You may substitute any simple object for the O or the bar, provided that the object is easy for you to imagine. Do these mental exercises frequently so long as they are easy for you to do.

Night Blindness

In addition to doing the regular Bates program outlined in Chapter 6, add these special exercises.

1. Palm thoroughly outdoors in the dark, then practice seeing silhouettes of trees, rooftops, etc. To practice this, keep your head moving, doing vertical and horizontal or circular swings. Night vision depends on the rods located on the sides—not the center—of the retina, and because you must use peripheral, rather than

central, vision, movement is absolutely essential to good night vision. Check also to see whether you are Vitamin A deficient because Vitamin A aids the rods. But since Vitamin A is one of the vitamins that can be toxic if taken in large doses, consult your doctor or nutritionist as to the amount you can safely take.

2. Place pieces of white paper of various sizes on a table. Sit nearby in the dark and palm, then swing across the table. Practice this a lot; your vision will improve with practice. Be sure to swing your head. Again you will be seeing peripherally, not centrally, so looking directly at the paper will be of no avail. It takes 20 to 30 minutes to become completely accustomed to darkness, so palm for this initial time.

3. Stand on a dark street and look at a headlight or streetlight, blinking and breathing. Now turn your back on the light and note houses and silhouettes of other objects by swinging across them. Close your eyes and rest often.

Color Blindness

Everyone is colorblind in the absence of light or in very dim light. At dawn and dusk, objects all appear to be various shades of gray and black. And though most people with defective vision retain the ability to distinguish colors to some degree, the sharpness of colors disappears; as they improve their vision, one of the first things they notice is the brightness of various colors. Even glasses change color tones slightly. It takes normal, rested eyes to see color as it exists in nature.

Color blindness is a misnomer because few people fail to see any colors at all. Most color blindness consists of an inability to distinguish between red and green, although other confusions exist. Color blindness can be eased, however, by relaxation and education. In fact, primitive man apparently was color blind because the retinal nerves were not developed enough for him to notice differences in the colors caused by light rays thrown off an object. Gradually, humans acquired this sensitivity.

Even today there are differences in how people perceive various colors—mostly the tertiary colors. The differences are the result of culture and environment. Different languages have words for colors that do not exist in other languages; these are colors of slight tonal variations not considered significant in other cultures. The Eskimos, for example, live most of the year in a white world of snow. Just as they perceive different kinds of snow and have words for these various kinds of snow, they also perceive different tones of white that are important enough for them to name. If the human race through the ages acquired an ability to distinguish colors, and if today peoples of different cultures perceive some colors differently, why should an individual suffering from minor color blindness not be able to do so as well?

Color is the breaking-up of light into its component wave lengths, which the eye then sees as the various colors. An object seems to be a particular color because it reflects certain wavelengths of light and absorbs all the others. We see only the reflected light. Color in light and color in pigment act differently. In light, if all the colors of the light spectrum are combined, the result is white; in paint pigment, such a mixture results in a dirty brown-black.

As any elementary schoolchild knows, there are three primary colors—red, blue, and yellow. They are called primary because they cannot be obtained by mixing other colors; they simply exist. But these are also the three colors that, in the course of evolution, the retinal nerves first learned to dinstinguish. The secondary colors—orange, purple, and green—are formed by mixing the primaries: red + yellow = orange; red + blue = purple; blue + yellow = green. In addition, there are complementary colors: red and green; yellow and purple; blue and orange. When complementary colors are used together, they are restful to the eyes. If, for example, you were to look intently at a red object for a few minutes, then close your eyes, you would see its complement, green; if you looked at green, you would see red. The same is true of the other two sets of complementary colors.

Red, yellow, and orange are warm colors; blue, green, and purple are cool. These two classes of colors function differently. Cool colors seem to recede, convey a feeling of lightness, and are restful. Warm colors appear to advance, convey a sensation of heaviness, and are stimulating. Cool colors are pain absorbing. Green, for example, is used to take pain out of burns.

Colors also react differently in relation to one another and in different levels of light. On the color wheel, neighboring colors—for example, yellow and green, or yellow and orange—accent each other; complements tend to dull each other. Colors also appear different in different light and at different distances. As distance increases, or the intensity of light diminishes, color dims until the point where everyone is blind to color. Color blindness may occur at one distance and not at another, in shade and not in sun, or vice versa. All of these points are important for the person working on regaining color sensitivity.

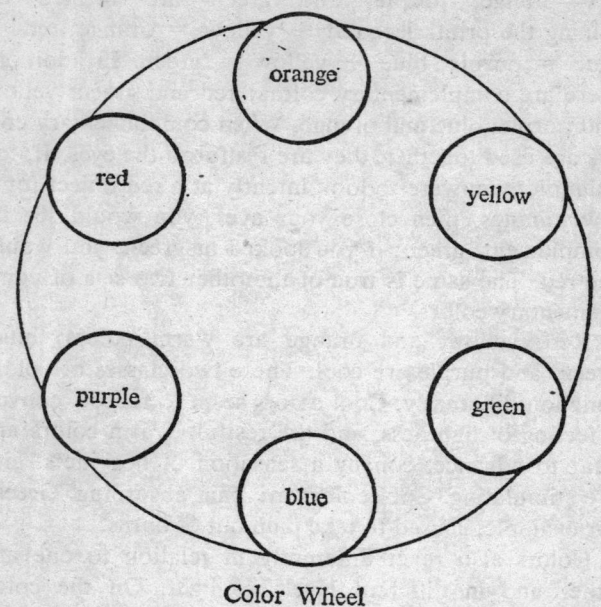

Color Wheel

Fatigue is also a factor. It is important that you discover where and when you are color blind, and to which colors. Your eye doctor and your own observations, and the verifications of friends or family, will help you to know your weaknesses.

Bates taught that all cases of color blindness could be normalized by sunning, centralization, palming, and swings, particularly the mental swings. The habit of staring must be broken, and shifting via the swings and relaxation helps alleviate the problem.

Work through the 12-week vision program, adding these color exercises as you proceed with the regular exercises before you work with color. Always work each eye individually with color, as well as both together, and change distances, and from sun to shade to artificial light.

It is also advisable to take Vitamin A supplements. Vitamin A promotes growth and development of protective tissues, including the tissue linings of the nose, throat, and eyes. Since the retina is an inner lining of the eye, it benefits. Vitamin A apparently also affects the cones of the retina, and it is the cones that perceive color. Because Vitamin A is toxic in amounts that are too large, be sure to consult your doctor or nutritionist about the amount you should take.

Color Lessons

Beginning with Lesson 1 of the regular program, do a color lesson with every lesson. And work in daylight, if at all possible, rather than artificial light. But gradually, over the weeks, do the color exercises in all kinds of lighting—sun, shade, and artificial light. For the first week, work four to five days in the sun and shade and the last two to three days in artificial light as well, *if* it is easy for you to do so. If not—i.e., if the colors become indistinct in one type of light and not another, always work in the light easiest for you until working in the other types of light becomes easier.

1. With a small watercolor set that contains the three primary colors, make squares, about 3" x 3", of red, yellow and blue, using only enough water to lift the paint, so that your colors are strong and bright. Paint on white paper and have a friend with good color perception help you identify and, later, mix the colors. When your squares are dry, use your nose to swing and circle the red square. Then close your eyes, take a deep breath, and imagine the red square. Open your eyes and swing the red square again. Do this five or six times, then do the same exercise with the blue and yel-

low squares. Become familiar with these three colors; *feel* the differences between them.

2. Mix equal amounts of red and yellow to get orange; blue and yellow to get green; blue and red to get purple; and paint another square of each color. Repeat the above exercise with the orange, green, and purple squares. Label all six squares on the back with the name of the color. Frequently flip through the squares, naming them until you do not need to look on the back for the correct name. Continue doing these two activities as long as necessary, and be sure to work with your paint set daily, even if only for a short time.

3. On a large piece of white paper, paint circles of the six colors, filling them in entirely. Label the colors and put them on the order as illustrated below.

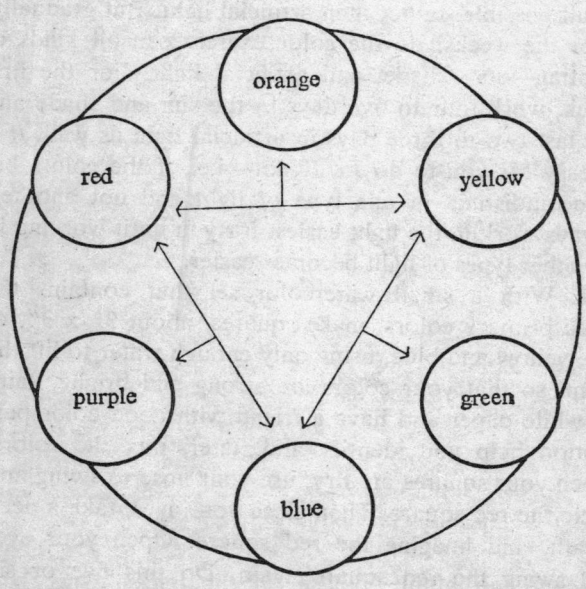

On another piece of paper, paint bands of red, blue, yellow, and red again. Make the bands about two inches wide and four inches long, and leave about two inches of white space between them. Swing on each color, noticing and feeling the differences between them. When the primes are dry, mix your three secondary colors and paint them between the two primes that are used to produce them. Be sure to have your colors

red	orange	yellow	green	blue	purple	red

verified. Then label these. Cut an inch off the bottoms of the bands and arrange the colors according to their order in the rainbow.

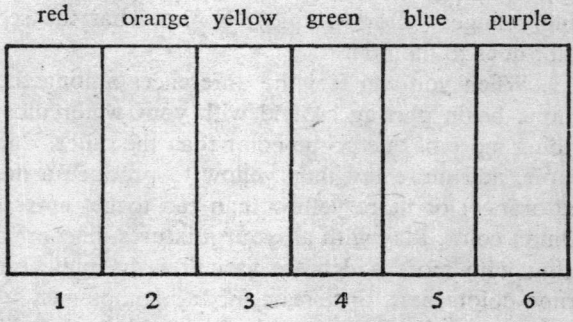

Label and number these on the backs. Carry them around with you and frequently practice with them, lining them up in order. Soon you will not need to look at the back to verify the color.

4. Search for pictures in magazines that match up with your colored swatches. Compare them for intensity of hue. Cut out examples of your six colors, and start collecting examples of both lighter and deeper shades of each color. Again, be sure you get your choices verified.

5. Notice natural objects that belong to each color. Mentally verbalize the color with the object, as, for example, red rose, orange orange, yellow squash. Green leaf, blue sky, purple eggplant.

6. Go to shops and department stores with someone who can help you find and verify objects that match your colors, or are the same tones as those colors.

7. Collect beads, pegs, yarns, etc., and match them up with your color squares.

8. Work with colors in various combinations, trying to *feel* the differences and similarities between them. Place a warm color (red, orange, yellow) beside a cool one (blue, green, purple) and feel the difference. Place two warm colors and two cool colors side by side; place the colors next to their complements (red/green; blue/orange; yellow/purple). Notice what the second color does to the first.

9. When you can feel the differences among the six colors, begin playing around with your watercolor set, adding more of one prime color than the other. For example, add more red than yellow to produce a deeper red-orange; or more yellow than red to get more of a salmon color. Play with all your mixtures, becoming familiar with more and more variations in hue. Use the prime colors first, then start mixing complements: red with green; yellow with purple; blue with orange. Use a lot of the prime, a little of the complement and observe what happens. Play with the colors; enjoy yourself. Use

the activities outlined above to find objects that match these new colors you are producing. Remember to stop if you get tired or bored. Rest often and, as with everything else, blink, breathe, and swing.

Other Disorders

While other serious disorders can be eased with the Bates method, if you are a sufferer of, for example, iritis, retinitis pigmentosa, blindness, color blindness, etc., it is advisable that you work with an experienced Bates teacher who will, no doubt, also want to work closely with a willing ophthalmologist. To work on your own might be harmful if you do not do the exercises with relaxation, and under such conditions relaxation can be difficult to achieve by yourself. A Bates teacher can be located by contacting the Bates-Corbett Teachers' Association, 11303 Meadow View Road, El Cajon, California 92020.

CHAPTER 9
Working with children

Bates suspected that some vision disorders, myopia particularly, were not so much hereditary as *catching*—that the eyes of the parents communicated strain to the young child, who, as a great imitator, picked up the external "look" of myopia, gradually achieving the inner strain as well. Such an interpretation may account more than heredity does for the frequency with which bespectacled parents engender bespectacled children.

Weak vision may develop very early on or later, during the school years, but the school years certainly create an atmosphere conducive to the development of poor vision or to the worsening of already existing conditions. Prior to the school years, a child is not accountable for what he sees. In play, the child may or may not see all objects well at all times, but this is of little consequence. One child may say, "Look at that butterfly!" His nearsighted playmate looks up, cannot see it, and simply returns to whatever is occupying him. It does not matter that he cannot see it. In school, however, his not seeing the blackboard has relatively serious consequences. The teacher may point to some numbers on the board and ask Johnny to give the sum. Johnny strains, squints, and cannot make out the numbers. The teacher is waiting, his classmates are watching, the pressure builds. Shame or embarrassment are the result, and from that day forth, fear is established in Johnny, a fear out of which he develops a habit of eyestrain, and it causes his vision to go from bad to worse.

Parents should periodically check their youngster's vision by casually asking questions about objects at different distances. Often this procedure is more successful than taking the child to a doctor because many young children are frightened by doctors and the strange environment and equipment.

Prevention

All children's vision can be helped by swinging them as infants. To swing, hold the child facing out in front of you, and rock him from side to side, or rock in a rocking chair. The motion is beneficial in two ways: first, it promotes relaxation in both infant and parent; second, it will cause the child's eyes to shift as you swing back and forth. The parent's relaxation is as significant as the child's. Too often, in our hurried, harried lives, parental attention to children is accompanied by tension; this tension transmits itself to the child in the subtle body communication between child and parent. Often it happens that when a busy, tense parent hands over an angry, tense child to another, more disinterested adult—a grandparent or friend—the child visibly and quickly relaxes, settles down, and falls asleep. Tension is insidious and affects all of our being—mind, emotions, and body. The first step for both parent and child is to create times of relaxation.

To sun a youngster's eyes, swing him, head tilted back, to catch the sun full on his closed lids. His eyes will close in the bright light, and while some children may at first react against the bright light, recoiling from it as if in pain, the combination of light and warmth and the gentle rocking motion will soon bring about the desired end. Sun only a few minutes, then move to the shade and continue to swing. An older child can be taught to swing and sun alongside his parent. The joint activity will be a source of pleasure to him as long as the parent keeps the period short and makes it a happy activity. Done frequently, such swinging and sunning can go a long way to prevent poor vision.

Even a nervous child can be induced to palm for five to ten minutes if the palming period follows sunning and swinging and is accompanied by a pleasant story. Bedtime or naptime is a good time for a child to palm. And stories that are continued from day to day create anticipation, making the activity one he will look forward to. Be aware of your child's stresses, and do not expect him to do visual work when he is upset or distressed any more than you would expect him to eat a big dinner when he is in such a condition. And *never force* any of the activities. Find a time when he is alert and happy, and *ready*. To interrupt a game, for example, is not recommended, as it will cause the child to resent the vision games.

Perhaps the best way to prevent any physical disorder—visual or otherwise—is to promote a loving, pleasant environment. Those few words make it sound so easy, but discovering what makes for your child's sense of love and comfort is the art of parenting, and no one can teach you but yourself and your child. Your desire to achieve this, along with your own sensitivity, will be your best guides, though general child-rearing practices can be used as a basis. Above all, do not *worry* about your child's eyes, or make him concerned about seeing. One of the first steps in developing poor vision is a person's loss of belief that he *can* see well.

Correction

Any of the exercises described in this book can be used to correct a child's visual disorder, provided they are done for one short period per day—20 minutes at the most—and provided the child has *fun* doing them. If you feel anxious or impatient with him, the exercises will be of little value. Get him *playing, laughing* and *enjoying* himself. This can require a lot of patience and ingenuity on your part.

Infants and children up to four years of age will benefit simply by daily sunning, palming, and swinging, as described in the section above. Even when a child's eyes are out of line, the exercises can be beneficial by allowing the child to relax the large muscles, which then communicate their relaxation to the smaller and involuntary muscles. Given such a rest, eye muscles that pull one or both eyes out of focus may straighten. With daily practice in the art of relaxation, these muscles will strengthen and hold. Be careful, however, in your enthusiasm and desire to help the child, that you do not overdo it by lengthening the time period so that he tires or becomes bored, or by having more than one or two of these periods per day. If the child begins to resist your overzealousness, you will have lost whatever gains he might have made.

For children over four years of age, here is a sample lesson you can work out with them.

1. Sunning

Stand beside the child, facing the sun. Morning or late afternoon, when the sun is low in the sky, are the best times. Both of you should close your eyes and swing slightly from side to side, turning your heads so that the sun "travels" from cheek to cheek. Sing a sun or morning song—any song—as this not only establishes a rhythm, but causes deep breathing, which further promotes relaxation as well as increases blood circulation. If possible, work outdoors; if not, work at a window or, if no sun is available, use the sunning lamp described in Lesson 1 of the Bates lessons. Call the child's attention to the way the sun moves from one side of his face to the other, gently caressing his eyes as it travels. After a minute of this, continue the movement but have him cover first one eye, then the other, with his palm so that he stimulates each eye individually. Be sure he does not press his hand against his eye but simply rests his palm over it without pressure. Finish sunning on both closed eyes. To end with one eye covered will cause discomfort, since the pupil of the palmed eye will be more enlarged than that of the uncovered one. No more than two to three minutes should be taken to do the whole sunning exercise.

2. Swings

a. The long swing. Teach him this swing, as described in Lesson 2 of the regular lessons. Again, sing along with the swing, or do it to music so that a rhythm is established. If your child is nervous, it might be best to take a brisk walk (brisk for him, not for you) or play some running or chasing games before the lesson so that he can release some of his tension. The long swing exercises his large muscles and relaxes him with its large, rocking motion. Relaxed, the child's eyes will begin to shift naturally. Swing for at least 100 swings.

b. The elephant swing is a variation of the long swing and can be substituted for it, or done in addition to it. Your child should stand the same way as for the long swing, but grasp his two hands together to form the elephant's trunk. He should bend over from the waist and rock from one side to the other, swinging his trunk. He can also do this swing as he walks around.

c. A further variation that young children love is the bag of gold swing. Here an adult with a good, strong back should stand behind the child and hold him around his middle. The child should go limp, bending from the waist, letting his weight fall on the adult's supporting arms. His feet and arms will hang free while the adult swings him gently from side to side, letting the ground flow smoothly past his gaze. This swing loosens up the tight muscles of the neck and spine, as well as allowing the eye muscles to let go. Children will sometimes do their own version of this swing, by hanging limply over a sling-type playground swing and then gently swinging back and forth.

After sunning and swinging, a child is usually ready to palm, although a more nervous child may need coaxing and even then be willing to palm for only a few minutes. Farsighted children and children with unfocused eyes are particularly susceptible to nervousness and do not take easily to palming. The nearsighted adult and child always enjoy palming because it is of the same world—the pulled-in, subjective world—that the myope has already created for himself by pulling his vision in close. But the farsighted child, whose inclination is to "keep an eye on things" out there, may feel threatened by being held in close behind his palms. Be aware of his anxiety, and be gentle about his palming. Let it be short, and keep him happy with a brief, pleasant story, preferably one that is continued from one palming period to another so he will look forward to the palming period in order to find out what is going to happen next. And rather than interrupt your child's play with others, turn the palming period into a group time. All

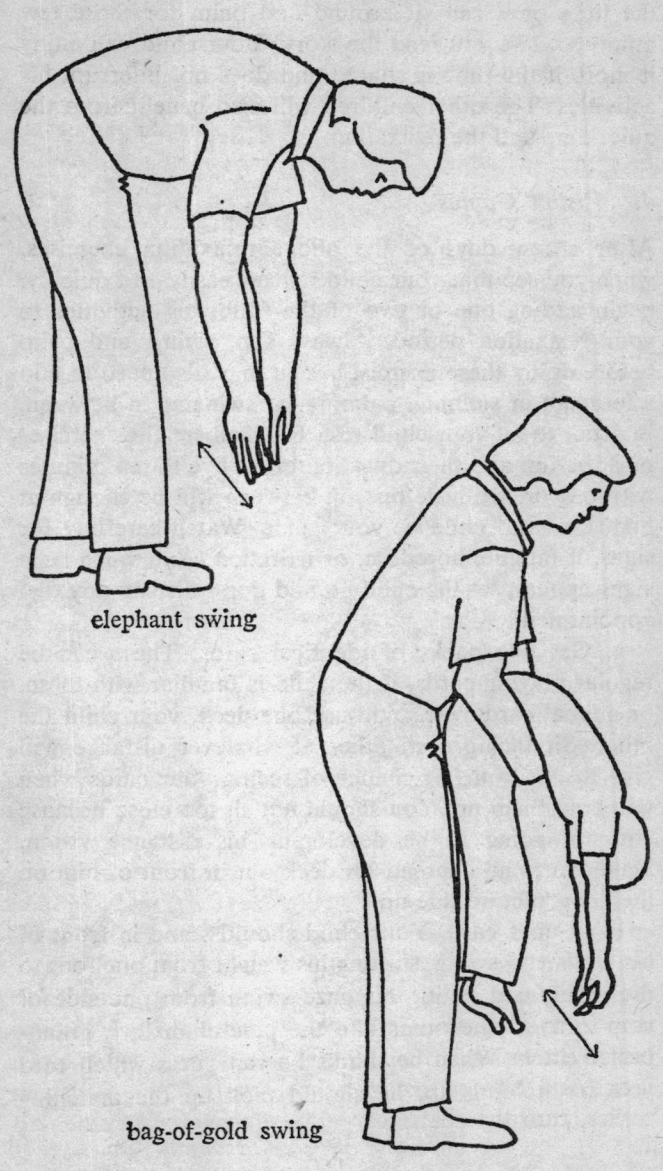

elephant swing

bag-of-gold swing

the little ones can sit around and palm for those few minutes while you read the story. Your child will enjoy it more if the time is shared and does not interrupt his activities. The other children will also benefit from the quiet time and the relaxation.

4. Vision Games

After a few days of the above relaxation exercises, when you see that your child relaxes easily and quickly, begin adding one or two of the following activities to your relaxation period. Always sun, swing, and palm before doing these exercises. You may also need to add a moment of sunning, palming, or swinging in between, in order to let your child rest. Remember: the exercises must be fun and their duration brief; five to ten minutes with one or two little rests in between will be enough at first. Let your child be your guide. Watch carefully for signs of fatigue, boredom, or irritation. And when such signs appear, let the child go and don't display any disappointment.

a. Get two packs of identical cards. These can be regular playing cards, if the child is familiar with these, or animal cards, etc. You use one deck, your child the other. Sit facing each other at whatever distance will give the child a fair chance of seeing your cards when you hold them up. You should not sit too close because you are going to be developing his distance vision. Have your child spread his deck out in front of him on the floor, picture side up.

Hold up a card. Your child should stand in front of his cards and swing, shifting his weight from one foot to the other, and letting his gaze swing from one side of your card to the other like the pendulum in a grandfather clock. When he thinks he can guess which card you are holding up, he should pick up the matching card from his deck and hold it up. If he guesses the right card, he runs across to you and "wins" your card, gaining one point. If he guesses the wrong card, he runs to you with his card, which you then win, along with a point. The run will help to relax him. Encourage him to really guess, and sit just far enough away so that he has a chance to win. Be sure he swings his gaze across your card; otherwise, he will stare or strain, thereby defeating the purpose of the game. If you notice strain, move closer. Play this game about three times a week. As he gets quickier in recognizing the cards, and winning, gradually move back to increase the distance between you. Use different decks of cards to provide variety.

b. Tie a weight—a bead, marble, nail, or whatever—to the end of a brightly colored piece of string or yarn. Sit near your child, facing him, and swing the weight like a pendulum, making a tick-tock noise to accompany the swinging. Now have your child palm his eyes, resting his elbows on his knees or on a table, and imagine the pendulum in its swing, following the movement from side to side with his nose. After 15 to 20 such swings, have him swing up the string to your hand, in his imagination, and call out the names of your five fingers, pointing his nose to each finger as he names it. You can give your fingers whatever names will be easy for him to remember. When he has named your fingers, he should run his nose back down the string and do another 15 to 20 tick-tock swings with the pendulum. This exercise is restful and can be used as a brief rest period during the card game.

c. Play follow the bee. Sit opposite your child, and hold a small ball of yellow yarn—the bee—between your fingers. Tell your child to follow the bee with his nose. Then, making a buzzing sound, loop the bee up, down, and around, moving in close and away from your child. Dive-bomb his nose; have fun with it.

d. Play ball, again emphasizing that your child follow the ball with his nose. The game can be catch or chase or roll-on-the-ground, depending upon your child's dexterity.

Use your imagination to invent your own vision games and activities. Any fast-moving game is good, as long as it follows the rule for children: *fun* and *brief*. Let your child play that he is an airplane or dance a sailor dance as he swings from side to side. In short, enjoy the activities and stop them before he gets tired. Always practice with your child when he is alert, not when he is tired or thinking of food. Remember: if you are bored, he will be too.

In working with a child with squint, it will probably be best (though not absolutely necessary) to get a Bates teacher, or at least a friend, to help him. Squint children are highly nervous and irritable, thus irritating. Never punish such a child during vision work. He cannot help his behavior. Distract him; help him to have a good time, to laugh. Sing songs and act them out; play follow the leader, with *you* always being the leader.

Read the section on ambliopia and squint, and always employ directional swings—swings that pull your child's eye in the correct direction—opposite to the way his eye pulls, whether in or out, or up or down.

The mirror swing is especially good in working with squint children. Patch the stronger eye, and have your child do the long swing with a mirror set up directly behind him. Each time, as he swings toward the mirror, he is to glance into it with the unpatched eye. Be sure his glance favors the direction in which you want to pull the weaker eye. For example, if his right eye turns in, patch the left, and have him glance into the mirror over his right shoulder as he swings to the right. If the right eye pulls outward, he should glance into the mirror over

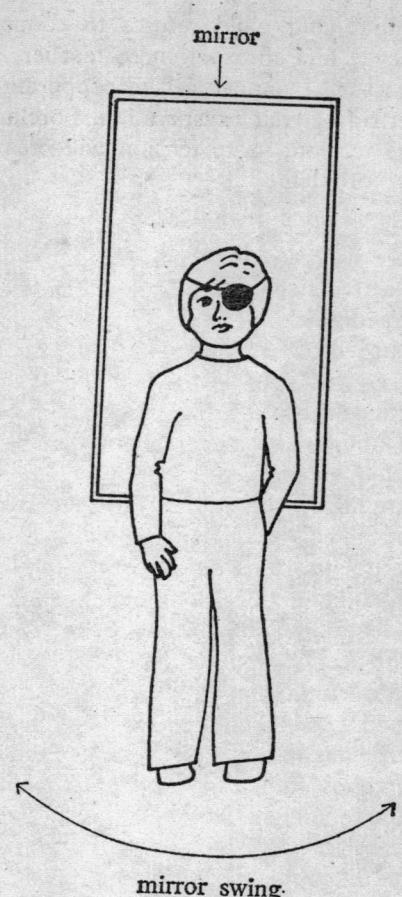

mirror swing.

his left shoulder across his nose. If the left eye is the weaker, reverse the above directions to the exercise.

Be aware of your own parental feelings and expectations, regardless of the condition of your child's vision. If you cannot remain relaxed, if you feel angry or disappointed that your child refuses to cooperate, then stop. Either get him an experienced teacher, or give up on the project until you can get his cooperation or until you can get rid of your exasperation. Forcing him will create more tension; more tension will create a more severe vision problem.

CHAPTER 10
The Bates laws of vision

The following 11 "laws" are included as food for thought. Some of them are quite obvious, others at first seem hidden, or mysterious, later to become clear as you work on your vision.

1. The shorter the shift, the greater the relaxation.

2. Imperfect sight results when there is an effort to see.

3. Anything you do to get vision is the wrong thing.

4. The secret of vision is mental relaxation. The secret of mental relaxation is memory.

5. The eye sees best only at the point regarded, or vision is imperfect.

6. The point regarded changes, moving rapidly and continuously.

7. As the point regarded changes, the object regarded appears to move in the opposite direction.

8. The normal eye blinks easily, automatically, and often.

9. We can only see what we can imagine. We can only imagine what we can remember.

10. The normal eye sees well in bright, dim, or artificial light, but sees best in bright sunlight.

11. Palming is the most important way to rest the eyes.